start
fresh!

start fresh!

YOUR COMPLETE GUIDE TO *Midlifestyle* FOOD AND FITNESS

CHEF AND DOCTOR ON THE RUN

Diane Clement and Dr. Doug Clement

Foreword by Pat Quinn

whitecap

Edited by Ann-Marie Metten
Proofread by Joan E. Templeton and Lesley Cameron
Design by Michelle Mayne
Food photography by Shawn Taylor
Food styling by Jennifer Stamper
Cover photo and additional author photos by Tina Graham
Exercise photos by Michelle Mayne

Printed in Canada by Friesens

LIBRARY AND ARCHIVES CANADA CATALOGUING IN PUBLICATION

Clement, Doug
     Start fresh! : your complete guide to midlifestyle food and
fitness / Doug Clement, Diane Clement.

Includes index.
ISBN 978-1-55285-919-3

     1. Middle-aged persons—Health and hygiene. 2. Middle-aged
persons—Nutrition. 3. Physical fitness for middle-aged persons.
I. Clement, Diane, 1936- II. Title.

RA777.5.C54 2008   613'.0434   C2007-905571-0

The publisher acknowledges the financial support of the Government of Canada
through the Book Publishing Industry Development Program (BPIDP) and the
Province of British Columbia through the Book Publishing Tax Credit.

To our grandchildren–Lucia Clement, Max Clement-Gale and Coco Clement. You are the future.

To their parents, Jennifer Clement and Vincent Gale, and Rand Clement and Suzanne Campbell Clement.

To our high-spirited Clement and Matheson clans.

To our patriarch, Uncle Maurice Clement, who is now 98 years young. Along with your wife, Patricia, you've set an example of a healthy lifestyle that spurs the next generation on to live life to its fullest.

Contents

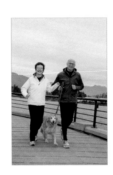
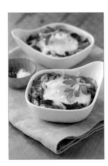

Foreword

Start Fresh! is a practical guide to achieving a better quality of life. Although Doug and Diane Clement are addressing all baby boomers—there are so many of us midlifers who are stuck in habits that negatively affect our health—they could be speaking directly to me.

I once made my living as a professional athlete. I thought I was invincible and that health problems happened to other people, not to me. I ate and drank anything I wanted to, but I assumed that my high level of physical activity automatically assured my good health. And it did . . . for a time. When I retired as a professional National Hockey League (NHL) player and began my professional coaching career, my physical activity was greatly diminished, but my eating and lifestyle habits didn't change at all.

In 2002, I was diagnosed with a heart condition that was aggravated by overworking, poor eating habits and not enough exercise. So I started to take the steps toward healthy living—by eating right and exercising regularly. And I got results. The change has been dramatic. Six years after that considerable health scare, I am finally experiencing health in my mid-60s. Unfortunately I had to have a crash before I started taking control and making better lifestyle choices. But you don't have to wait. It's never too late to start fresh.

The book cites four practical lifestyle choices that we all need to make if we are to live productive, independent and healthy lives as we age: maintaining proper body weight and waist size; eating more fruits and vegetables; exercising regularly; and not smoking. These are common-sense rules to live by, but I didn't pay attention to any of it. And I wasn't alone. A recent study found that less than 10% of those surveyed practice these habits (see page 2).

Why listen to Doug and Diane? Don't just listen to them because they were world-class athletes, or because they coached and treated top athletes. Don't just listen to them because Doug taught and practiced medicine and Diane became an award-winning author of health-conscious cookbooks. And don't just heed their advice because what they say makes sense, and can make a difference in our lives if we take control.

Listen to Doug and Diane because they are living proof that a healthy lifestyle helps you achieve *vigor, clarity and independence* (as they put it). They'll motivate you to take action by looking at the reasons why you need to pay attention to your health, and help you understand why you may not be exercising and eating healthily.

First, take a hard look at your lifestyle by creating your "HealthSpan report card" (Doug shows you how on pages 8–15). Second, learn how easy it is to get moving. It is proven that people of all ages can improve the quality of their lives through a practice of moderated activity. Doug attacks your excuses by showing you how to exercise and how to work fitness into your schedules. Third, win the war on the waist. Diane shares how a combination of fitness and healthy eating is necessary, and she provides 7 steps to eating right for life as well as helps us shop, plan menus and entertain. She then proceeds to give us page after page of wonderful recipes. Although moderation has never been a big part of my vocabulary (I'm a meat-and-potatoes guy), I'm looking forward to trying out all these delicious dishes.

Doug and Diane's wisdom, which they have earned over many years of work, study and personal experience, can motivate you to start fresh too.

Pat Quinn

Acknowledgments

A special thank you to: Arnold Gosewich, our book agent and friend, whose guidance, wisdom and expertise over these many years are truly appreciated. Michael Burch, owner of Whitecap Books, for having faith in our book. Robert McCullough, publisher of Whitecap Books, whose passion is food. We've had many fun times doing cooking events with Robert and our dear friend Caren McSherry, cookbook author and owner of The Gourmet Warehouse in Vancouver. When Robert suggested Doug and I do a lifestyle book for Whitecap Books we were delighted. Managing editor Taryn Boyd's and Robert's expertise and creative efforts made our life easier in giving birth to *Start Fresh!* Ann-Marie Metten, our editor, who carefully steered and molded *Start Fresh!* with patience and excitement. Michelle Mayne, Whitecap's art director, who was a delight to work with on our photo shoot. Shawn Taylor, our expert food photographer, who brought life to every food presentation. Jennifer Stamper, our talented food stylist, who kept us busy as we whipped up the many dishes for the photo shoots. To our family and friends who were our tasting team. Their enthusiasm was our reward.

Introduction

THE BOOK

This book aims to guide people in midlife who are stuck in habits that affect their good health.

An overabundance of food combined with increasing limitations on physical activity not only contribute to our growing overweight but also push us into the negative consequences of diabetes, high blood pressure, high cholesterol and heart attack. Physical activity has disappeared from the workplace today and the BlackBerry has extended our stressful workdays. We reduce physical activity while facebook.com flourishes.

And we're eating more. Today's fast food portion sizes have tripled in caloric value from 50 years ago. The calorie content in a serving of French fries has moved from 200 to 570 calories, providing an extra 370 calories that need to be burned off, perhaps with 4 or 5 miles (about 1 hour) of walking. Are you doing that?

We passed through midlife decades ago. We found that aging is very real and we found it necessary to adapt our lifestyle to fit the changes in our bodies. We would like to share our experience with you and motivate you with a reality check, and then with a plan for manageable exercise and healthy eating.

In the first chapter, we look at the reasons you may not be exercising now and help you understand how getting active can actually solve some of the problems that may be holding you back.

In the second chapter we ask you to take a hard look at your lifestyle. We assess aspects of your life to create what we call your HealthSpan report card. It should give you an accurate idea of how healthy you are right now.

To help you improve your health, in the third chapter Doug prescribes 4 fitness plans that will gradually and effectively help you meet your good health goal.

In the fourth chapter, Diane guides you through day-to-day menu planning and helps you keep to a healthy eating plan even while entertaining guests on the weekend. Diane expertly provides nearly 100 healthy recipes that will tempt your palate and tease your taste buds while offering healthy food choices that taste and look great.

Together we hope that our passion for food, fitness and fun will be the first step, and you will catch the spirit. It could change your life.

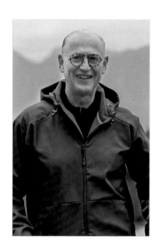

THE DOCTOR

Little did we know that a Sunday run around Victoria's Beacon Hill Park would redirect our lives so profoundly. I was 45 years of age and a lifelong runner. I had just run my first marathon 2 weeks before. As an advocate of the exercise and health movement, physician, coach and Olympic athlete, I was the "picture of health."

Suddenly my comfortable easy-paced run began to feel like a climb up Mount Everest. My chest started pounding and I became short of breath. I was unable to keep up with my running partners. Shortly after returning to Vancouver, I found myself in St. Paul's Hospital undergoing electrocardioversion (shocking the heart to correct an irregular heartbeat). My mortality was showing for the first time.

After that Sunday in 1979 my heart irregularity recurred only occasionally, maybe 3 or 4 times a year. For 24 hours, I would have a rapid, irregular heartbeat, anxiety, dizziness and shortness of breath. The rest of the time, I was fully able to work and exercise.

Then things changed rapidly. On May 17, 1998, I collapsed early on a Sunday morning, falling suddenly to the floor with violent, disabling vertigo and vomiting—symptoms of a stroke. I was unable to stand and it took nearly an hour to inch upstairs on my back and awaken Diane for help.

After almost 2 weeks in hospital, I came home to the task of learning to walk and move. Fortunately I had no cognitive loss or paralysis but I was like a 10-month-old baby taking his first tentative steps. At physiotherapy, I spent hours relearning control of movement.

Progression was rapid and I was determined to participate in the Longest Day Run on June 21. Just 5 weeks after the stroke, our daughter, Jennifer, and I ran the 5 kilometers in 24 minutes and 55 seconds.

Our brains and bodies have an amazing ability to change and regroup if we demand they do so.

THE CHEF

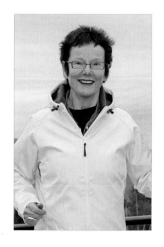

It was a wake-up call for me when Doug started having heart problems in his 40s. Another jolt of reality came when Doug watched while I was lining up ingredients in our kitchen to teach a cooking class with Julia Child's inspired recipes, which are laden with butter and cream, and asked "Diane, who are you killing tonight?" That was the moment of truth for me. We can't eat Christmas dinner every day.

The challenge for me as a chef was to create recipes for a new cookbook with less fat, less sugar and less salt. In 1986, our *Chef and Doctor on the Run* lifestyle cookbook was launched. It became a Canadian bestseller, addressing the balance of food and fitness. Now, 22 years later, we combine healthy eating with a balance of exercise to help the millions of North Americans at midlife who want to restore balance in their lives and regain health.

Where does the balance lie? How do we find the right approach to health, nutrition and exercise, which varies for each and every one of us? It depends on how active we are, but it also depends on our age and our genetic history. It's a balancing act for life for all of us. The facts are that if we truly want a realistic balance of healthy eating and exercise, then each one of us has to take responsibility for achieving it. No one can give it to us.

IF A PROPER
LIFESTYLE WERE
A PILL, THEN
YOU WOULD
PAY PLENTY FOR
A PRESCRIPTION.
WHY WOULD
YOU NOT DO
IT WHEN THE
TOOLS ARE
AVAILABLE AT
NO COST?

on your marks!

Adopting a healthy lifestyle now can add years to your life and give you the good health you need to enjoy them. Life expectancy has increased dramatically in the past century by an incredible 33 years–from 47 years in 1900 to 80 years today. Many of us have watched our parents and grandparents live longer but develop health conditions that rob them of the freedom to enjoy an active and independent life.

As a result, baby boomers no longer graciously accept declining physical and mental powers as an inevitable part of growing older. We want to live with vigor, clarity and independence.

Instead of thinking about the number of years we live—our "lifespan"—we need to begin to think about the quality with which we live our lives. The number of years we enjoy productive activity, independence, freedom of choice and good health could be called our "HealthSpan." In part, the length of our HealthSpan depends on our genetic makeup. But an active life and a healthy diet can work together to overcome the limitations of our genetics.

Proof that exercise can improve your quality of life

Research has shown that changes in our lifestyle can produce positive changes in our longevity. King reported in the *American Journal of Medicine* in 2007 the results of a study of more than 15,000 adults aged 45 to 50. Adherence to the following 4 lifestyle habits was assessed:

1 maintaining proper body weight and waist size
2 eating 5 or more fruits and vegetables daily
3 exercising regularly
4 not smoking

Only 8.5% of these middle-aged Americans practiced these habits at the outset of the study. Are you in that minority? What's your excuse?

The vital part of this study was revealed in the 4-year follow-up. The group who newly adopted positive lifestyle habits at midlife had a 35% decrease in cardiovascular disease and a 40% reduction in mortality.

Do you maintain proper body weight and have an ideal waist size? Do you eat the recommended number of fruit and vegetables every day? What's your excuse?

The Mayo Clinic has summarized the benefits of adequate physical activity as follows:

» helps to manage body weight
» combats chronic illness, including cardiovascular disease, hypertension, diabetes mellitus, osteoporosis and some forms of cancer
» improves mood
» strengthens heart, lungs and muscles
» promotes healthy sleep
» produces inherent enjoyment (exercise is fun)

Are you exercising to optimize your health? What's your excuse?

One more habit that needs to change: medical studies are conclusive that addiction to nicotine promotes an early death. Yet 25% of North Americans still smoke. Are you in that group? Why?

We've heard all your excuses:

» I don't have time.
» I'm too tired.
» I feel self-conscious.
» It's boring.
» I'm not an athlete.
» I've failed before.
» I'm afraid of injury and pain.

Have you heard of determination, persistence, originality, problem-solving and a never-give-up attitude? Excuses are not solutions.

To get past the excuses and establish healthy habits, a change of thinking needs to factor into the good health equation. You have total control of the healthy choices you make every day. Begin by making gradual changes in the amount of exercise you do each day and in your food intake. Soon healthy choices will become a habit and you'll maintain good health for years to come.

Exercise can improve your mood

Dr. Kristen Vickers-Douglas, a psychologist at the Mayo Clinic, reported that even small amounts of physical exercise can help to reduce symptoms of both depression and anxiety. Regular exercise does the following:

» stimulates mood-enhancing neurotransmitters in the brain
» improves sleep
» eases muscle tension
» reduces levels of the stress hormone cortisol
» increases body temperature, which may calm the body and mind

People who experience clinical depression can benefit from exercise if, with the advice of their doctor, they take part in an activity they love and set reasonable goals.

Delays are to be expected and should be accepted as a part of the process of getting fit. If you don't manage to get out and exercise for a couple of days, it doesn't mean you can never exercise again. Just get back at it and gradually you will find that a vigorous bout of exercise can improve your mood.

Chronic pain and exercise

A patient came to our sports medicine clinic with severe chronic pain in both heels. She had been confined to a wheelchair for more than a year. She had seen doctors at two university hospitals in Western Canada with no solutions found after weeks of testing. She was unable to work and was desperate with suicidal thoughts as she lost ground in this battle with chronic pain. She felt fearful and depressed over her uncertain future.

Our initial assessment recognized that this patient had an uncommon inflammatory condition called bilateral plantar fasciitis. Our experience allowed us to reassure her that she would make a complete recovery if she followed our rehabilitation plan.

The problem was that she was caught in a vicious cycle of inactivity, amplifying her pain and promoting further inactivity. Her system was getting weaker and weaker as she met pain with continued immobility. She was told to record her pain and activity level in a daily log and to send it to me weekly. The strategy was to slowly and progressively increase small doses of non-weight-bearing exercise that would not amplify her current level of pain. Initially she cycled on a stationary bike with no tension for 30 seconds and added 30 seconds each day. She was told that her current level of pain would not disappear but nor would it worsen. The goal was to gradually increase her level of function until she was able to stimulate and rebuild the scarred tissue in the plantar fascia (arch of the foot) under each heel. She was told to expect that this could take many months of exercise on her part.

After 2 months she was cycling for 1 hour. Resistance was added gradually to the stationary bike; then she began weight-bearing exercise—first in the pool to reduce her body weight and then on land. Just 3 steps of walking were introduced and this was increased by 3 steps over subsequent days. A strengthening program using toe raises and heel drop exercises was gradually introduced.

Her daily charts initially reinforced her progress in her exercise loading but after several months her pain charting on the 0 to 10 scale revealed a steady but gradual decline. The painful scar in the plantar fascia was modified by her effort to allow full range of motion and painless standing and walking. Her vigor and outlook normalized as her function returned and she resumed work and daily life.

This example shows that chronic pain responds to small doses of progressive resistance exercise. Many painful degenerative arthritic conditions of the back respond to static V-sit exercises (page 32) and knees respond to a squat program (page 33). The same applies to painful tendon inflammations in a variety of locations in the body.

Great ways to work fitness into your schedule

If you've tried but failed, look at your failure as an opportunity to find different ways to solve the problem. Try one approach and, if that doesn't work, try, try and try again! Temporary delays to success can be met with a variety of solutions:

CARPE TEMPUS! SEIZE YOUR TIME

» Exercise in 10-minute sessions several times throughout the day. They all add up.
» Get up 30 minutes earlier and exercise first thing in the morning.
» Make exercise a priority and schedule it into your day.
» Walk or cycle to work, or park farther away from your destination.
» Plan weekend activities with family or friends that involve hiking, cycling or swimming.

DON'T BE BORED! HAVE FUN

» Choose an activity you love.
» Do lots of different activities: dance, climb, ski and walk.
» Find friends who like the same activity.
» Enroll in a fitness class or join a sports club.

GET OVER FEELING SELF-CONSCIOUS

» Exercise in the privacy of your own home.
» Choose an activity that suits your level of conditioning.
» Find or create a group of people who feel self-conscious, too, and exercise with them.

FIND YOUR INNER ATHLETE

» Everybody has an activity that suits his or her physical abilities.
» Find the program that suits your body.
» Focus on improving your physical skills.

FAILED MEANS DELAYED, NOT FINISHED

» Start slowly and gradually.
» Substitute patience for aggression.
» Expect that setbacks will be part of reaching your goal.

IF YOU'RE FEELING TIRED, IT'S TIME TO REVITALIZE

» Expending energy builds stamina and ultimately increases energy.
» Appropriate exercise is guaranteed to improve your mood.
» A group or partner will kickstart your plan.

IF PAIN IS A PROBLEM, GET STRONG

» A slow and progressive exercise program may actually relieve chronic pain.
» Start with micro doses of exercise in segments as short as 30 seconds. Increase duration by 30 seconds each day.
» Exercise increases muscle strength and shock absorption.
» Increased strength enhances body alignment and prevents further injury.

"THE BEST SIX DOCTORS
ANYWHERE AND
NO ONE CAN DENY IT
ARE SUNSHINE, WATER,
REST AND AIR,
EXERCISE AND DIET.
THE SIX WILL GLADLY
YOU ATTEND
IF ONLY
YOU ARE WILLING
YOUR MIND WILL EASE
YOUR WILL THEY'LL MEND
AND CHARGE YOU
NOT A SHILLING."

–Nursery rhyme quoted by Wayne Fields
in What the River Knows, 1990

get
set!

Before you begin to make changes in the amount of exercise you do each day and in your food intake, let's figure out how healthy you are right now. Here are 7 questions to assess your current lifestyle and provide you with feedback on how your lifestyle stacks up against the ideal. The answers all fit into what we call your HealthSpan report card. It assesses your lifestyle, weight, functional age and life expectancy and can help you understand that you need to make a fresh start.

1   Are you carrying too much weight?
YOUR BODY MASS INDEX

Let's begin with the main concern for a lot of people: how much you weigh. Better than stepping on the scale, a good tool for determining your health risk is to assess your body mass index or BMI. It classifies you as underweight, at your ideal weight, overweight or obese.

To calculate your BMI, you need to measure your height and weight and then do some mathematical calculations. You can do this yourself if mathematics is a passion or you can use an online BMI calculator, which automatically does it for you. There's a good online BMI calculator on the US Centers for Disease Control website (www.cdc.gov). Look under Tools & Resources near the bottom right of the website home page to find the BMI Calculator.

If you're keen to do the math yourself, use the following formula:

> **BMI = (weight in pounds x 703) / (height in inches x height in inches)**
>   *or*
> **BMI = weight in kilos / (height in meters x height in meters)**

You are underweight if your result is below 18.5.
You are at your ideal weight if your result is between 18.5 and 24.9.
You are overweight if your result is between 25 and 29.9.
You are obese if your result is over 30.

You can see that the BMI helps identify overweight and obesity. A high BMI is one indication of increased risk of developing overweight- or obesity-related diseases such as heart disease, hypertension and diabetes. If you're overweight it's risky; if you're obese it's dangerous!

As an example, let's use my height and weight to calculate my BMI. I stand 5 foot 10.5 inches tall and weigh 171 pounds. My BMI calculation would be as follows:

BMI = (171 pounds x 703) / (70.5 inches x 70.5 inches)
BMI = 120,213 / 4,970.25
BMI = 24.1

With a BMI of 24.1, I am on the borderline of being overweight. If my weight balloons up just a few pounds, I enter the danger zone of being overweight, with a BMI over 25. That's an incentive for me to monitor my weight, food intake and exercise.

On the other hand, Diane stands 5 foot 5.5 inches tall and weighs 141 pounds. She has a BMI of 23.1, well within the ideal range.

WHAT IS YOUR BMI? MY BMI IS   .

Are you overweight? Do you need to start fresh?

2   *Are you shaped like an apple or a pear?*
YOUR WAIST-TO-HEIGHT RATIO

Another indicator of increased risk of developing overweight- or obesity-related diseases is your waist circumference. Measuring your waist and comparing it to your height is another effective way to assess your risk for the health complications of being overweight or obese.

The math here is much simpler. Simply:

> **Divide your waist measurement in inches or centimeters by your height in inches or centimeters.**

The ideal is below 50%.

For example, my waist measures 36 inches and I stand 5 foot 10.5 inches tall; Diane's waist measures 32 inches and she's 5 feet 5.5 inches tall.

FOR DOUG   Waist-to-height ratio = 36 inches / 70.5 inches = 51%
FOR DIANE   Waist-to-height ratio = 32 inches / 65.5 = 49.2%

You can see that Diane is in the safe zone while I'm at risk of developing heart disease, hypertension and diabetes. I either have to grow a few inches taller (not likely) or, more realistically, reduce my waist size by about an inch.

WHAT IS YOUR WAIST-TO-HEIGHT RATIO?
MY WAIST-TO-HEIGHT RATIO IS   .

Do you need to grow an inch or more?

3 *Is your middle too big?*
YOUR WAIST MEASUREMENT

A third screening test for overweight- and obesity-related disease is even more direct.

Just measure your waist in inches or centimeters.

To measure your waist, stand with your abdominal muscles relaxed. Breathe out and wrap the measuring tape around your waist, level with the highest portion of your pelvic bone. The tape measure should be horizontal to the floor.

You are at risk:
If your waist measures more than 37 inches (94 cm) for men.
If your waist measures more than 31.5 inches (80 cm) for women.

You are in the danger zone:
If your waist measures more than 40 inches (100 cm) for men.
If your waist measures more than 35 inches (88 cm) for women.

Diaz of the University of Leicester found that the incidence of diabetes was not predicted as accurately in non-Caucasian ethnic groups with BMI results as compared to a combination of waist circumference and height-to-weight ratio.

Lear at Simon Fraser University found that BMI results in the Chinese and South Asian population underestimated visceral adipose tissue and recommended the inclusion of waist circumference and height-to-weight ratios. He suggested that 35 inches should be the upper limit of normal for men of Asian descent.

Determining abdominal obesity using this waist measurement combined with BMI produces an accurate assessment of an impending metabolic syndrome. This was supported by research done at San Diego State University by Misra and his co-workers.

Metabolic syndrome is defined as abdominal obesity combined with 2 of the 4 following criteria:

1   increase in the fat level in your blood (higher plasma triglycerides)
2   decrease in high-density lipoproteins (HDL, the good cholesterol)
3   higher blood sugar (the prediabetic state)
4   hypertension (increased blood pressure)

Metabolic syndrome is a strong predictor of impending heart disease, stroke and type 2 diabetes. For us, we are close to the at-risk category with our waist measurements.

WHAT IS YOUR WAIST CIRCUMFERENCE?
MY WAIST CIRCUMFERENCE IS   .

4 *Are you younger than you think?*
THE REALAGE CALCULATOR

The RealAge calculator is a patented series of online questions that estimate the biological age of your body, your RealAge, compared to your chronological age. The questions assess your medical and family history and then help you evaluate aspects of your lifestyle. Your pattern of exposure to tobacco, alcohol, stress, nutrition and fitness are calculated to either increase or decrease your functional age.

> **The RealAge calculator can be used online without charge but the website does include advertising. Access the Internet site at www.realage.com.**

After I completed the online questions, my results calculated my BMI at 24.1, my calendar age at 74 years and my RealAge at 64.9 years. Diane's results showed a BMI of 23.1, her calendar age at 71 years and her Real-Age of 63.2 years. In other words we can enjoy living with the vigor of a couple almost a decade younger than our chronological ages.

WHAT IS YOUR REALAGE SCORE? MY REALAGE SCORE IS   .
Are you above or below your chronological age?

5 *When is your turn coming?*
LIFE EXPECTANCY ESTIMATE

A variety of online calculators similar to RealAge are available, all with the goal of estimating your life expectancy. When using each calculator, you generally complete a questionnaire that probes your current and past medical history and assesses your lifestyle.

We tried the online calculator of Dean P. Foster, a professor in the department of statistics at the University of Pennsylvania posted at http://gosset.wharton.upenn.edu/mortality/. Other online life-expectancy questionnaires are available on insurance company websites. Check out Metropolitan Life's calculator on the Retirement page of the website at www.metlife.com. Northwestern Mutual Life also hosts a longevity calculator on the Learning Center page of their website at www.nmfn.com.

Our results suggested a life expectancy of 91 years for me and of 94 years for Diane. This suggests we could live almost another 20 years beyond our current ages. We like this forecast for obvious reasons.

Clearly none of these estimates can predict the future with any real certainty but the process may well act as a motivator to make changes in your current lifestyle or reinforce maintaining your current direction. It's an incentive to stay on course!

WHAT IS YOUR ESTIMATE OF LIFE EXPECTANCY?
MY LIFE EXPECTANCY IS   .

Do you need to change some lifestyle habits?

6   *How much food is enough?*

YOUR BASAL METABOLIC RATE

We are what we eat. If we only ate as much as the total calories we used, then we'd never gain an ounce!

How much food do we really need to eat? The answer is surprisingly simple: if total calories consumed equal total calories burned, then total body weight remains constant. If calories consumed are greater than calories metabolized, then body weight increases.

Metabolic rate is dictated by our bodies, which seek stability (homeostasis) so that they can maintain a constant internal environment and still accommodate a level of physical activity. The body burns calories to maintain our internal temperature, help our organs function and regenerate cellular tissue. The rate at which our bodies burn calories is known as our basal metabolic rate (BMR). It's the energy cost of keeping the body functioning at rest. In addition to this basal rate, energy is required to move the body in physical action during work and play. The demand for this caloric energy varies based on our level of physical activity.

To help you find balance between your food intake and your physical output, first calculate your personal BMR, and then use your BMR to calculate how many calories you need to eat depending on how much you exercise. The formula is as follows:

Caloric cost of BMR + Caloric cost of physical activity = Total Caloric Need

If Total Caloric Intake equals Total Caloric Need, then body weight remains constant. If Total Caloric Intake exceeds Total Caloric Need, then body weight increases. If Total Caloric Intake is less than Total Caloric Need, then body weight decreases.

You can calculate your personal BMR using the Harris-Benedict Equation:

FOR MEN: BMR = 66 + (6.23 x weight in pounds) + (12.7 x height in inches) - (6.8 x age in years)

FOR WOMEN: BMR = 655 + (4.35 x weight in pounds) + (4.7 x height in inches) - (4.7 x age in years)

or

FOR MEN: BMR = 66 + (13.7 x weight in kilos) + (5 x height in centimeters) - (6.8 x age in years)

FOR WOMEN: BMR = 655 + (9.6 x weight in kilos) + (1.8 x height in centimeters) - (4.7 x age in years)

or

Use the online calculator at www.bmi-calculator.net/bmr-calculator/.

When Diane and I entered our height and weight and then our ages, the online calculator came up with the following results:

DOUG'S (THE DOCTOR'S) BMR is 1,523 calories daily.
DIANE'S (THE CHEF'S) BMR is 1,242 calories daily.

With our BMR in hand, the next step is to find out how many calories we can consume according to how much exercise we do, as follows:

SEDENTARY (no or very little exercise) = BMR x 1.2
LIGHT ACTIVITY (exercise 2 days each week) = BMR x 1.375
MODERATE ACTIVITY (exercise 4 days each week) = BMR x 1.5
HIGH ACTIVITY (exercise more than 6 days each week) = BMR x 1.7

We estimate that we fit into the moderate activity category because we try to work out at least 4 days per week. Our formula looked like this:

BMR x 1.5 = Total Caloric Intake
THE DOCTOR   1523 x 1.5 = 2,284 calories daily
THE CHEF   1242 x 1.5 = 1,863 calories daily

The health consequences of overweight and obesity

Overweight and obese individuals are at increased risk for many diseases and health conditions, including the following:

» hypertension
» high cholesterol, low HDL cholesterol, or high levels of triglycerides
» type 2 diabetes
» heart disease
» stroke
» gallbladder disease
» osteoarthritis
» sleep apnea and respiratory problems
» some cancers (endometrial, breast and colon)

SOURCE: US CENTERS FOR DISEASE CONTROL AND PREVENTION

The UK Department of Health Estimated Average Intake for women is 1,940 calories and 2,550 calories for men. Surprisingly, the US Centres for Disease Control and Prevention Dietary Guidelines are 1,833 calories for women and 2,475 calories for men. These caloric intakes are for people of average size and average activity levels. When calculating your daily caloric intake, remember: who is average?

WHAT IS YOUR BMR? MY BMR IS   .

Do you need to exercise more because you love to eat?

7   *The Naked Truth!*

YOUR HEALTHSPAN REPORT CARD

You've now calculated your BMI, waist-to-height ratio, waist measurement, RealAge, life expectancy and total caloric need. Let's pull all these statistical results together to create a HealthSpan report card.

Here's what our HealthSpan report cards look like:

DOUG
The Doctor
> **BMI** 24.1 *Ideal*
> **WAIST-TO-HEIGHT RATIO** 51% *At risk*
> **WAIST** 36 inches *On the border*
> **REALAGE** 64.9 years *9.1 years younger than chronological age*
> **LIFE EXPECTANCY** 91 years *Higher life expectancy than average*
> **TOTAL CALORIC INTAKE** 2,284 calories *Below average*

DIANE
The Chef
> **BMI** 23.1 *Ideal*
> **WAIST-TO-HEIGHT RATIO** 49.2% *Ideal*
> **WAIST** 32 inches *On the border*
> **REALAGE** 63.2 years *6.8 years younger than chronological age*
> **LIFE EXPECTANCY** 94 years *Higher life expectancy than average*
> **TOTAL CALORIC INTAKE** 1,863 calories *Near average*

What Is Your HealthSpan Report Card?

BMI
Underweight ☐   *Ideal* ☐   *Overweight* ☐   *Obese* ☐

WAIST-TO-HEIGHT RATIO
Ideal ☐   *At Risk* ☐   *Danger Zone* ☐

WAIST
Ideal ☐   *At Risk* ☐   *Danger Zone* ☐

REALAGE
Younger ☐   *Older* ☐   *than your chronological age*

LIFE EXPECTANCY
Lower ☐   *Higher* ☐   *than average*

TOTAL CALORIC INTAKE NEED
Lower ☐   *Higher* ☐   *than average*

You can compare our results with yours and with the ideal. If you find that your results are perfect, then congratulations! You're obviously on the right track. Perhaps this book will increase your knowledge and inspire you to continue to make great health choices.

If your results are not ideal and you want to find out what to do about it, then keep reading. Start fresh now!

"I HAVE TWO
DOCTORS, MY
LEFT LEG AND
MY RIGHT."

–G.M. Trevelyan

go!

THE DOCTOR SHOWS YOU HOW TO GET FIT

Your HealthSpan report card gives you a good idea of whether your lifestyle is on track or whether you need a fresh start. These figures do not lie. Your results give you an objective review of your current lifestyle and predict the risks that lie ahead. You can improve your fitness level by changing obvious habits.

You can cease smoking if you're currently hooked on nicotine. You can limit your use of alcohol. You can eat better by increasing the number of fresh fruits and vegetables you eat and limiting the number of processed foods you eat. You can also get active.

Here we present 4 training programs to lead you into the world of physical activity. They include weight training that can be done at home or at the gym. On alternate days you could power walk or run. For some people, other types of activities will be better choices. Your best choice may depend on your body type and your age.

FITNESS VARIES WITH BODY SHAPE

When you look around you, you'll see a range of body types—from the short and slight (called ectomorphs), to the medium-tall and heavily muscled (called mesomorphs), to the tall and fat (called endomorphs).

From my experience as a coach in track and field, I've found that people with different body types tend to succeed in the physical activity that suits their physical attributes. For example:

» *marathoners* are usually short and slight (they're ectomorphic, sort of like Formula 1 racing cars)
» *sprinters* are usually medium height and have powerful musculature (they're mesomorphic, sort of like drag racing cars)
» *shot putters* are usually tall and extremely heavy in build (they're endomorphic, sort of like Kenworth trucks)

These athletes are at the peak of fitness in their own disciplines, and each has found a sport that suits their body type.

The way we look and the way our muscles are able to perform is based on a genetic code passed through the generations. This range of body types is actually more complex than I have outlined here, as ectomorphs can also be thin and tall (well suited to basketball), mesomorphs can also be muscular and short (well suited to wrestling) and endomorphs can also be heavy and have a medium build (well suited to football linebackers). All possess great fitness but it's specific to their tasks. We each possess a blend of body type traits. Our genetic background, our nutritional intake and our level of physical activity create body type.

The significance of this observation is that each of us should tailor our choice of fitness activity to our passions but also to our body profile. Those of us with endomorphic traits may well find non-weight-bearing activities such as swimming and cycling easier, while those with ectomorphic characteristics might find running distances easier for them.

Follow your heart when choosing the activity you want to do. You can choose activities ranging from dance, tai chi, yoga, walking, climbing, skateboarding, skiing, hiking and running to martial arts, golf, swimming, cycling, racquet sports and team sports. Just make movement part of your daily routine. If you choose an activity that's easy to do because it suits your body type, you'll find it easier to give your fitness and health a high priority.

THE KEY: BURN 600 CALORIES EVERY DAY

Physical activity is important because it helps balance the difference between the caloric need of our basal metabolic rate and the number of calories we eat each day. If basal metabolic rate is 1,500 calories and our recommended daily caloric intake is 2,100 calories, then we have 600 calories that need to be used by physical activity.

The goal of burning 600 calories every day may seem hard to reach. How do you spend time on your personal fitness program and still meet the needs of work and the family? Remember that every step you take contributes to your total activity for the day. Every step counts, so combine the energy burned in all activities you have done during the day to reach your goal.

Try to build movement into all your other daily activities. Getting out of your car is a good place to start. Commuting requires and can accommodate more walking if you park several blocks away from your destination or choose public transportation, which often includes walking to the transit stop or running when you're late for the bus.

More ideas: use stairs instead of elevators. Walk during your lunch break. Make family activities physical by walking, hiking or skiing together. Use every opportunity to move and groove through each day so that it's easy to burn your 600-calorie target.

3 sample fitness prescriptions

To show you how to work fitness into your daily habits, here are 3 examples of people at various levels of fitness and different stages of midlife. We evaluate their HealthSpan report card and then prescribe a fitness plan that blends strength and endurance programs.

The changes we suggest create a deficit of 300 to 600 or more calories each day. We set a modest goal of creating a 1,000-calorie deficit each

Walking works

Every step you take is important. Remember the following:
» Walking can help you achieve your fitness goals.
» Aim to walk 10,000 steps per day.
» Try to walk in natural settings.
» Outfit yourself with weather-proof clothing.
» Wear sturdy, comfortable walking shoes.
» Consider joining a walking or hiking group in your same age group.

Most important, incorporate walking into the activities you love. For example, bird watching involves long walks in natural settings. Golfing involves walks between holes.

Many pursuits include moderate physical activity. Build walking into the pursuit of your passions and you'll fall in love with the act of walking itself.

PACE	% OF MAXIMUM HEART RATE	BEATS PER MINUTE (BPM)
Easy pace	less than 60%	90 to 105 bpm
Brisk pace	60% to 70%	105 to 123 bpm
Fast pace	greater than 70%	120 to 140 bpm

week, accumulating to a 3,500-calorie deficit each month.

By burning more calories than you take in—in this case, up to 3,500 calories per month—you draw on your energy stores sufficiently to burn 1 pound of body fat each month. Do this for 1 year and you have a 12-pound loss of fat and a reduced waist size. Or, if your weight and waist size are already ideal, burn more calories than you take in and you can eat the big, gooey chocolate dessert that's been calling your name! Make these changes permanent by increasing the duration and intensity of your exercise and by paying more attention to your food choices. Your HealthSpan report will gradually improve.

By creating hypothetical HealthSpan report cards and then offering exercise solutions that fit easily into daily life, we trust that you will see the benefits of increased exercise and healthy eating. We want to inspire you to get active and eat healthy, too.

EXERCISE PRESCRIPTION A: BACK IN THE RUNNING

You're a male, 55 years of age in apparent good health. You stand 5 feet, 9 inches tall and notice that your trousers seem tight around the waist at 190 pounds. You exercise occasionally, maybe once or twice a week.

HEALTHSPAN REPORT CARD

BMI 28.1 *Overweight*

WAIST-TO-HEIGHT RATIO 55% *At risk*

WAIST 38 inches *At risk*

REALAGE 57 years *You are older than your chronological age*

LIFE EXPECTANCY 68 years *You have a lower-than-average life expectancy*

These HealthSpan results indicate that your lifestyle urgently needs a makeover.

After consulting your health care provider, you choose to return to running, which you did regularly more than 20 years ago. You also decide to use the gym close to your place of work. Your program will involve exercise 6 days each week, with 3 alternate days in the HealthSpan 10K Walk Run Program (page 23) and 3 alternate days on the PowerFit Gym Strength Program (page 37). You'll rest on the seventh day.

EXERCISE PRESCRIPTION B: WORKING OUT AT HOME

You're a female, 48 years of age, stand 5 feet, 4 inches tall and weigh 165 pounds. You're currently inactive but used to play basketball in high school.

HEALTHSPAN REPORT CARD

BMI 28.3 *Overweight*

WAIST-TO-HEIGHT RATIO 57% *At risk*

WAIST 36 inches *At risk*

REALAGE 49 years *You are older than your chronological age*

LIFE EXPECTANCY 71 years *You have a lower-than-average life expectancy*

These HealthSpan results suggest that your lifestyle needs to start fresh.

After consulting your health care provider, you choose to walk more but you need an incentive. You decide to become involved in an annual 10K charity walk and to use the distances and time required as a training goal. You also are prepared to do strength workouts at home because you don't have access to a gym. Your exercise program will involve a time commitment of 6 days a week with 3 alternate days in the HealthSpan 10K Power Walk Program (page 25) and 3 alternate days in the PowerFit Home Strength Program (page 32). These are followed by 1 day's rest.

EXERCISE PRESCRIPTION C: CYCLING TO SAFETY

You're a male, 65 years of age, you stand 6 feet, 1 inch tall and you weigh 265 pounds. You have no regular physical activities but are keen to become active. You played football in college.

HEALTHSPAN REPORT CARD

BMI 35 *Obese*

WAIST-TO-HEIGHT RATIO 58% *At risk*

WAIST 42 inches *Danger Zone*

REALAGE 59 years *You are older than your chronological age*

LIFE EXPECTANCY 74 years *You have a lower-than-average life expectancy*

These HealthSpan results demand immediate intervention.

After consulting your health care provider, you choose to return to cycling, which you did regularly while in your 40s. You also decide to use the gym at the community center. Your program will involve exercise 6 days each week, with 3 alternate days in the cycle program that includes rides outdoors as well as indoors on recumbent and upright stationary bikes. The other 3 days you'll do the PowerFit Gym Strength Program (page 37), and on the seventh day you'll rest.

You decide to set a goal to participate in a charity cycle event that involves more than 2 hours of cycling. The event is scheduled to take place in 6 months so you develop a program that gradually builds to 2 hours of cycling.

During the first month, you start out with modest rides of 5 minutes at a moderate intensity. Over the next 3 weeks, you build the duration of your rides by 5 minutes each week. After 1 month you're riding 20 minutes 3 times a week. By the end of the third month, you're riding 60 minutes 3 times a week.

Over the next 3 months, you vary the length of your rides, with a short day, a medium day and a long day:

DAY 1	40 minutes
DAY 2	60 minutes
DAY 3	80 minutes

In months 4, 5 and 6, Days 1 and 2 remain at 40 minutes and 60 minutes but on Day 3, preferably when you're cycling outdoors, you increase your time by 5 minutes each week. This program would bring the long ride on the weekends to almost 2 hours, the duration of the target charity ride.

Training Programs

Here are the training programs that we prescribed in the sample exercise prescriptions. They offer a variety of options for fitness, from learning to run to power walking to strength training at the gym and circuit training at home. The 4 training programs are:

» HealthSpan 10K Walk Run Program helps you learn to run.
» HealthSpan 10K Power Walk Program helps you walk faster.
» PowerFit Home Strength Program shows you how to work out at home.
» PowerFit Gym Strength Program shows you what to do at the gym.

Each program requires between 30 minutes and 1 hour each day. Make them a habit by committing to a program for at least 6 months, and then build exercise into your early morning schedule or exercise at noon or after work. Gradually create time for exercise in your daily schedule and reinforce your success with incentives.

Keep a record of your training results. Weigh yourself at least once a week and record your weight. As you become more active you'll gain muscle mass that will eventually help to produce a healthy body weight. As you become fitter, the size of your waist measurement will be the most reliable indicator of success, not the weigh scale, which may not reflect your loss of fat. Reward yourself as you begin to see the results of your dedicated work.

These programs intensify gradually so don't leap ahead of the schedule. Stay on the program so that your body adapts slowly to the increasing exercise load. Always seek medical clearance from your physician before embarking on these programs.

HEALTHSPAN 10K WALK RUN PROGRAM

This 13-week training schedule will help beginners develop sufficient stamina and endurance to participate in a 10K community run. Organizations in many cities host community runs as fundraisers throughout the year. You can participate in these runs every couple of months if you gradually improve your fitness over the weeks before the first run and maintain a regular training schedule between runs. Begin your training by finding a run that you'd like to do and then working backward 13 weeks to find your starting point. Remember that the run portion should be very easy.

EQUIPMENT NEEDED

» Sweat suit and a good pair of running shoes
» Stopwatch
» Water bottle

	SESSION 1	SESSION 2	SESSION 3
WEEK 1	40 minutes Walk 5 minutes to warm up. Run ½ minute. Walk 4½ minutes. Do this 6 times. Walk 5 minutes to cool down.	40 minutes Walk 5 minutes to warm up. Run 1 minute. Walk 4 minutes. Do this 6 times. Walk 5 minutes to cool down.	40 minutes Walk 5 minutes to warm up. Run 1½ minutes. Walk 3½ minutes. Do this 6 times. Walk 5 minutes to cool down.
WEEK 2	40 minutes Walk 5 minutes to warm up. Run 2 minutes. Walk 3 minutes. Do this 6 times. Walk 5 minutes to cool down.	40 minutes Walk 5 minutes to warm up. Run 2½ minutes. Walk 2½ minutes. Do this 6 times. Walk 5 minutes to cool down.	40 minutes Walk 5 minutes to warm up. Run 3 minutes. Walk 2 minutes. Do this 6 times. Walk 5 minutes to cool down.
WEEK 3	40 minutes Walk 5 minutes to warm up. Run 3½ minutes. Walk 1½ minutes. Do this 6 times. Walk 5 minutes to cool down.	40 minutes Walk 5 minutes to warm up. Run 4 minutes. Walk 1 minute. Do this 6 times. Walk 5 minutes to cool down.	40 minutes Walk 5 minutes to warm up. Run 4½ minutes. Walk ½ minute. Do this 6 times. Walk 5 minutes to cool down.
WEEK 4	40 minutes Walk 5 minutes to warm up. Run 5 minutes. Walk 1 minute. Do this 5 times. Walk 5 minutes to cool down.	45 minutes Walk 5 minutes to warm up. Run 6 minutes. Walk 1 minute. Do this 5 times. Walk 5 minutes to cool down.	42 minutes Walk 5 minutes to warm up. Run 7 minutes. Walk 1 minute. Do this 4 times. Walk 5 minutes to cool down.

CHART CONTINUED ON NEXT PAGE

	SESSION 1	SESSION 2	SESSION 3
WEEK 5	**46 minutes** Walk 5 minutes to warm up. Run 8 minutes. Walk 1 minute. Do this 4 times. Walk 5 minutes to cool down.	**40 minutes** Walk 5 minutes to warm up. Run 9 minutes. Walk 1 minute. Do this 3 times. Walk 5 minutes to cool down.	**43 minutes** Walk 5 minutes to warm up. Run 10 minutes. Walk 1 minute. Do this 3 times. Walk 5 minutes to cool down.
WEEK 6	**46 minutes** Walk 5 minutes to warm up. Run 11 minutes. Walk 1 minute. Do this 3 times. Walk 5 minutes to cool down.	**49 minutes** Walk 5 minutes to warm up. Run 12 minutes. Walk 1 minute. Do this 3 times. Walk 5 minutes to cool down.	**52 minutes** Walk 5 minutes to warm up. Run 13 minutes. Walk 1 minute. Do this 3 times. Walk 5 minutes to cool down.
WEEK 7	**55 minutes** Walk 5 minutes to warm up. Run 14 minutes. Walk 1 minute. Do this 3 times. Walk 5 minutes to cool down.	**58 minutes** Walk 5 minutes to warm up. Run 15 minutes. Walk 1 minute. Do this 3 times. Walk 5 minutes to cool down.	**61 minutes** Walk 5 minutes to warm up. Run 16 minutes. Walk 1 minute. Do this 3 times. Walk 5 minutes to cool down.
WEEK 8	**64 minutes** Walk 5 minutes to warm up. Run 17 minutes. Walk 1 minute. Do this 3 times. Walk 5 minutes to cool down.	**67 minutes** Walk 5 minutes to warm up. Run 18 minutes. Walk 1 minute. Do this 3 times. Walk 5 minutes to cool down.	**70 minutes** Walk 5 minutes to warm up. Run 19 minutes. Walk 1 minute. Do this 3 times. Walk 5 minutes to cool down.
WEEK 9	**55 minutes** Walk 5 minutes to warm up. Run 8 minutes. Walk 1 minute. Do this 5 times. Walk 5 minutes to cool down.	**54 minutes** Walk 5 minutes to warm up. Run 10 minutes. Walk 1 minute. Do this 4 times. Walk 5 minutes to cool down.	**58 minutes** Walk 5 minutes to warm up. Run 15 minutes. Walk 1 minute. Do this 3 times. Walk 5 minutes to cool down.
WEEK 10	**46 minutes** Walk 5 minutes to warm up. Run 5 minutes. Walk 1 minute. Do this 6 times. Walk 5 minutes to cool down.	**54 minutes** Walk 5 minutes to warm up. Run 10 minutes. Walk 1 minute. Do this 4 times. Walk 5 minutes to cool down.	**73 minutes** Walk 5 minutes to warm up. Run 20 minutes. Walk 1 minute. Do this 3 times. Walk 5 minutes to cool down.
WEEK 11	**50 minutes** Walk 5 minutes warm up. Run 3 minutes. Walk 2 minutes. Do this 8 times. Walk 5 minutes to cool down.	**46 minutes** Walk 5 minutes to warm up. Run 5 minutes. Walk 1 minute. Do this 6 times. Walk 5 minutes to cool down.	**58 minutes** Walk 5 minutes to warm up. Run 15 minutes. Walk 1 minute. Do this 3 times. Walk 5 minutes to cool down.
WEEK 12	**60 minutes** Walk 5 minutes to warm up. Run 50 minutes. Walk 5 minutes to cool down.	**43 minutes** Walk 5 minutes to warm up. Run 10 minutes. Walk 1 minute. Do this 3 times. Walk 5 minutes to cool down.	**52 minutes** Walk 5 minutes to warm up. Run 20 minutes. Walk 1 minute. Do this 2 times. Walk 5 minutes to cool down.
WEEK 13	**50 minutes** Walk 5 minutes to warm up. Run 40 minutes. Walk 5 minutes to cool down.	**30 minutes** Walk 5 minutes to warm up. Run 9 minutes. Walk 1 minute. Do this 2 times. Walk 5 minutes to cool down.	**Race Day** Rest for 2 full days before race day. Remember: do not use new shoes, socks or other gear on race day.

Maintain a pace schedule throughout your run by dividing the course into sections and pacing yourself throughout so that you're running each segment in the same amount of time. Start easy and use a watch to time your progress.

Good luck, and congratulations on completing your training and then on completing your run!

HEALTHSPAN 10K POWER WALK PROGRAM

Walking is an excellent form of exercise that improves cardiovascular and muscular fitness. For those who want to move faster than a stroll, here's a 13-week training program to follow. Whether you're a beginning walker or already an avid walker, this 10K Power Walk Program will provide you with a comfortable progression of distances and changes-of-pace to ensure your training is successful. You'll have variety and flexibility within the program to progress according to your own level.

Even though walking is the most natural exercise you can do, building up your distance and pace requires careful attention. Everyone's walking pace is different, but most adults at midlife walk at the following speeds:

» Easy pace equals greater than 16 minutes per mile (10 minutes per kilometer)
» Brisk pace equals 14 to 15 minutes per mile (9 minutes per kilometer)
» Fast pace equals less than 13 minutes per mile (8 minutes per kilometer)

Walking at an easy pace, you should able to carry on a conversation with a partner without effort. Walking at a brisk pace requires higher concentration, while walking at a fast pace demands total concentration.

One effective way of finding out the intensity of your walking is to use a heart rate monitor. As an option you can put your finger over the radial artery at your wrist and count the number of beats for 10 seconds; multiply by 6 to get your beats per minute. At what intensity are you walking? (See How fast are you walking? on page 20.)

The most direct and practical method for the beginner is to use your subjective sense of what is easy, brisk and fast for you. One important tip: work at a tempo well below your subjective guesstimate. Don't go too fast. Slow down and enjoy the scenery!

Each power walk session opens with a slow and easy walk to warm up and closes with a slow and easy walk to cool down. During most weeks, you'll increase the intensity of one session with intervals of brisk walking that alternate with 2-minute recovery intervals. Walking in intervals increases your body's capacity to carry oxygen and enhances the training effect. The other 2 sessions that week are walked at a steady pace for increasing periods of time. During these walks your personal pace is entirely up to you, and you should, for the most part, be relaxed, steady and able to carry on a conversation.

Remember to train on alternate days such as on Monday, Wednesday and Friday or on Tuesday, Thursday and Saturday. The recovery days could be either a complete rest or they could be used for easy cycling or strength training.

Choose courses that are natural with soft trails where possible. Be prepared for rain, wind and snow. Use a treadmill indoors when the weather is beastly. Remember to consult your health practitioner before embarking on any new exercise program. Consider joining a power walking group.

EQUIPMENT NEEDED
» Sweat suit and running shoes or casual clothes with comfortable shoes
» Stopwatch

	SESSION 1	SESSION 2	SESSION 3
WEEK 1	**44 minutes** Walk slow and easy for 10 minutes to warm up. Now walk briskly in intervals. Walk briskly 3 minutes. Walk slowly for 2 minutes in an easy recovery. Walk briskly 2 minutes. Walk slowly 2 minutes. Walk briskly 1 minute. Walk slowly 2 minutes. Repeat this combination once more. Walk slow and easy for 10 minutes to cool down.	**30 minutes** Walk slow and easy for 5 minutes to warm up. Walk for 20 minutes. Walk slow and easy for 5 minutes to cool down.	**35 minutes** Walk slow and easy for 5 minutes to warm up. Walk for 25 minutes. Walk slow and easy for 5 minutes to cool down.
WEEK 2	**40 minutes** Walk slow and easy for 10 minutes to warm up. Now walk briskly in intervals. Walk briskly for 2 minutes and then walk slowly for 2 minutes for an easy recovery. Repeat this combination 5 times. Walk slow and easy for 10 minutes to cool down.	**30 minutes** Walk slow and easy for 5 minutes to warm up. Walk for 20 minutes. Walk slow and easy for 5 minutes to cool down.	**40 minutes** Walk slow and easy for 5 minutes to warm up. Walk for 30 minutes. Walk slow and easy for 5 minutes to cool down.
WEEK 3	**54 minutes** Walk slow and easy for 15 minutes to warm up. Now walk briskly in intervals. Walk briskly 1 minute. Walk slowly for 2 minutes in an easy recovery. Repeat this combination 8 times. Walk slow and easy for 15 minutes to cool down.	**40 minutes** Walk slow and easy for 5 minutes to warm up. Walk for 30 minutes. Walk slow and easy for 5 minutes to cool down.	**50 minutes** Walk slow and easy for 5 minutes to warm up. Walk for 40 minutes. Walk slow and easy for 5 minutes to cool down.

	SESSION 1	SESSION 2	SESSION 3
WEEK 4 Easy Recovery Week	**40 minutes** Walk slow and easy for 10 minutes to warm up. Walk 20 minutes. Walk slow and easy for 10 minutes to cool down.	**30 minutes** Walk slow and easy for 5 minutes to warm up. Walk for 20 minutes. Walk slow and easy for 5 minutes to cool down.	**40 minutes** Walk slow and easy for 5 minutes to warm up. Walk for 30 minutes. Walk slow and easy for 5 minutes to cool down.
WEEK 5	**51 minutes** Walk slow and easy for 15 minutes to warm up. Now walk briskly in intervals. Walk briskly 5 minutes. Walk slowly for 2 minutes in an easy recovery. Repeat this combination 3 times. Walk slow and easy for 15 minutes to cool down.	**40 minutes** Walk slow and easy for 5 minutes to warm up. Walk for 30 minutes. Walk slow and easy for 5 minutes to cool down.	**50 minutes** Walk slow and easy for 5 minutes to warm up. Walk for 40 minutes. Walk slow and easy for 5 minutes to cool down.
WEEK 6	**66 minutes** Walk slow and easy for 15 minutes to warm up. Now walk briskly in intervals. Walk briskly 3 minutes. Walk slowly for 2 minutes in an easy recovery. Walk briskly 2 minutes. Walk slowly 2 minutes. Walk briskly 1 minute. Walk slowly 2 minutes. Repeat this combination 2 more times. Walk slow and easy for 15 minutes to cool down.	**40 minutes** Walk slow and easy for 5 minutes to warm up. Walk for 30 minutes. Walk slow and easy for 5 minutes to cool down.	**60 minutes** Walk slow and easy for 5 minutes to warm up. Walk 50 minutes. Walk slow and easy for 5 minutes to cool down.
WEEK 7 Over Halfway!	**5K distance, about 60 minutes** Walk slow and easy for 5 minutes to warm up. Walk 5 kilometers. You could carry a pedometer to measure the distance in kilometers. Or, before you run, ride 5 kilometers on your bike or drive the same distance in your car and follow the same course. Walk slow and easy for 5 minutes to cool down.	**50 minutes** Walk slow and easy for 5 minutes to warm up. Walk for 40 minutes. Walk slow and easy for 5 minutes to cool down.	**70 minutes** Walk slow and easy for 5 minutes to warm up. Walk for 60 minutes. Walk slow and easy for 5 minutes to cool down.
WEEK 8 Easy Recovery Week	**70 minutes** Walk slow and easy for 5 minutes to warm up. Walk for 60 minutes. Walk slow and easy for 5 minutes to cool down.	**30 minutes** Walk slow and easy for 5 minutes to warm up. Walk for 20 minutes. Walk slow and easy for 5 minutes to cool down.	**40 minutes** Walk slow and easy for 5 minutes to warm up. Walk for 30 minutes. Walk slow and easy for 5 minutes to cool down.
WEEK 9	**80 minutes** Walk slow and easy for 15 minutes to warm up. Now walk briskly in intervals. Walk briskly 5 minutes. Walk slowly for 2 minutes in an easy recovery. Walk briskly 4 minutes. Walk slowly 2 minutes. Walk briskly 3 minutes. Walk slowly 2 minutes. Walk briskly 2 minutes. Walk slowly 2 minutes. Walk briskly 1 minute. Walk slowly 2 minutes. Repeat this combination once more. Walk slow and easy for 15 minutes to cool down.	**50 minutes** Walk slow and easy for 5 minutes to warm up. Walk for 40 minutes. Walk slow and easy for 5 minutes to cool down.	**70 minutes** Walk slow and easy for 5 minutes to warm up. Walk for 60 minutes. Walk slow and easy for 5 minutes to cool down.

CHART CONTINUED ON NEXT PAGE

GO! « 27

	SESSION 1	SESSION 2	SESSION 3
WEEK 10	**80 minutes** Walk slow and easy for 20 minutes to warm up. Now walk briskly in intervals. Walk briskly 2 minutes. Walk slowly for 2 minutes in an easy recovery. Repeat this combination 10 times. Walk slow and easy for 20 minutes to cool down.	**50 minutes** Walk slow and easy for 5 minutes to warm up. Walk for 40 minutes. Walk slow and easy for 5 minutes to cool down.	**80 minutes** Walk slow and easy for 5 minutes to warm up. Walk for 70 minutes. Walk slow and easy for 5 minutes to cool down.
WEEK 11	**90 minutes** Walk slow and easy for 15 minutes to warm up. Now find a hill that has an incline of about 25 degrees. Walk briskly uphill for 1 minute and walk slowly back downhill at an easy recovery pace for 4 minutes. Repeat this combination 8 times. Using the same hill, walk briskly uphill for 30 seconds and walk slowly back down the hill at an easy recovery pace for 2 minutes. Repeat this combination 8 times. Or choose the no-hill option: walk briskly in intervals. Walk briskly 2 minutes. Walk slowly for 2 minutes in an easy recovery. Repeat this combination 10 times. Walk briskly 1 minute. Walk slowly 1 minute. Repeat this combination 10 times. Walk slow and easy for 15 minutes to cool down.	**50 minutes** Walk slow and easy for 5 minutes to warm up. Walk for 40 minutes. Walk slow and easy for 5 minutes to cool down.	**70 minutes** Walk slow and easy for 5 minutes to warm up. Walk for 60 minutes. Walk slow and easy for 5 minutes to cool down.
WEEK 12 Easy Recovery Week	**90 minutes** Walk slow and easy for 5 minutes to warm up. Walk for 80 minutes. Walk slow and easy for 5 minutes to cool down.	**50 minutes** Walk slow and easy for 5 minutes to warm up. Walk for 40 minutes. Walk slow and easy for 5 minutes to cool down.	**75 minutes** Walk slow and easy for 5 minutes to warm up. Walk for 65 minutes. Walk slow and easy for 5 minutes to cool down.
WEEK 13 This Is It!	**44 minutes** Walk slow and easy for 10 minutes to warm up. Now walk briskly in intervals. Walk briskly 3 minutes. Walk slowly for 2 minutes in an easy recovery. Walk briskly 2 minutes. Walk slowly 2 minutes. Walk briskly 1 minute. Walk slowly 2 minutes. Repeat this combination again. Walk slow and easy for 10 minutes to cool down.	**40 minutes** Walk slow and easy for 5 minutes to warm up. Walk for 30 minutes. Walk slow and easy for 5 minutes to cool down.	**Event Day 10K:** Maintain a steady pace throughout your walk by setting a pace schedule. Divide the course into sections and pace yourself throughout the walk so that you complete each segment in the same amount of time. Use a watch to follow your progress. Good luck and have fun.

The Sports Medicine Council of British Columbia derived this program from my Walk Run program by the InTraining Clinics organized by Lynn Kanuka, a medalist in the 3000 m at the 1984 Olympic Games. She was part of the training group of international runners that I had the privilege of coaching during the 1980s.

7 start fresh keys to help you get fit

My experience over the past 60 years, first as an athlete and later as a physician and coach, has given me the unique opportunity to see that common hazards need to be avoided when starting an exercise program. Being derailed by injury or overuse is a frustrating experience for all on the fitness trail. Grasp the following concepts and you'll keep on track.

1 TOO MUCH TOO SOON

Our initial enthusiasm to return to physical activity often wanes before we can feel the benefits of getting physical because of 2 common errors:

» We don't recognize that fitness is fleeting. We're not as strong or as fit as we thought we were.
» We get overtired or are injured because we're trying to do too much too soon.

Often we want to quit exercising because of the negative consequences of trying to train too hard and too soon. Enthusiasm seduces the individual into thinking: "The more work I do, the better I'll be." The reality is:

» The strength and endurance we once had can be regained. But strength and endurance are lost after 6 to 8 weeks of inactivity. Use it or lose it!
» An effective training program starts slowly and builds gradually.

Doing too much too soon can lead to failure to improve, fatigue and overuse injuries such as tendonitis and stress fractures to bones. These setbacks may cause a prolonged delay in training while you deal with the pain and other first symptoms of overuse injury.

A better approach is to seek the advice of a fitness professional who can guide you to an effective training program that starts slowly and builds gradually.

CONTINUED ON NEXT PAGE

What does it take to burn 600 calories?

You have a wide variety of activities to choose from. Here's how many minutes you need and how hard you need to work to burn 600 calories per day.*

EASY INTENSITY ACTIVITY

Easy intensity activity burns 4 to 6 calories every minute. You need 105 to 140 minutes of easy intensity activity to burn 600 calories. Keep it going this long to burn 600 calories:

Easy walking	140 minutes
Moderate walking	105 minutes
House-cleaning	105 minutes
Gardening	105 minutes
Tai chi	105 minutes
Yoga	105 minutes
Dancing	105 minutes
Easy rowing	105 minutes

*Calories consumed vary with the weight of the individual. These examples are for a 176 lb (80 kg) subject. A lighter person will burn fewer activities while doing the same activity for the same length of time and a heavier person will burn more calories.

What does it take to burn 600 calories?

MODERATE INTENSITY ACTIVITY

Moderate intensity activity burns 7 to 14 calories every minute. You need 50 to 90 minutes of moderate intensity activity to burn 600 calories. Keep it going this long to burn 600 calories:

Walking fast	90 minutes
Golfing while pulling a cart	90 minutes
Downhill skiing	90 minutes
Skating	80 minutes
Doing construction work	70 minutes
Hiking	70 minutes
Easy swimming	70 minutes
Easy cycling	70 minutes
Circuit weight training	50 minutes
Snowshoeing	50 minutes
Playing singles tennis	50 minutes
Swimming moderately	50 minutes
Easy running	50 minutes
Cycling moderately	50 minutes
Rowing moderately	50 minutes

2   THE NO BRAIN IN NO PAIN, NO GAIN

Some people think that we have to experience pain during exercise in order to gain fitness. This boot-camp mentality is probably the greatest barrier for people who are new to exercise and trying to launch themselves into fitness. Gradual introduction of exercise at an easy, comfortable pace is the best way to start. Beware of advice that comes from people with experience in combative sports such as hockey and football. And youthful instructors seldom have personal experience to advise the "mature student" in physical training. Instead, look for instruction from someone who has a background in dealing with individuals in your age group and at your fitness level.

3   ONE-TENTH RULE: YOUR BRAIN WILL FOOL YOU!

After meeting with more than 200,000 patients during 40 years of sports medicine practice, it became clear that, after a period of inactivity or injury, everyone overestimates their ability to exercise. Our miscalculation leads to renewed injury and failure to respond to training because the exercise load is damaging. That's why I devised the one-tenth rule. It says that slowly graduated loads of exercise should happen on alternate days, about 3 times per week.

The first time you exercise, you should do one-tenth of what you think you can do. For example, if you used to be active but haven't trained during the past 8 weeks, and you thought that 30 minutes of running would be about right, divide that target time by 10 and begin with 3 minutes. During your first week, you would run 3 minutes on Monday, 6 minutes on Wednesday and 9 minutes on Saturday. During the second week, you would continue increasing by one-tenth of your target running time per session, so that in week 2 you would run 12 minutes on Monday, 15 minutes on Wednesday and 18 minutes on Friday. In week 3 you would run 21 minutes on Monday, 24 minutes on Wednesday and 27 minutes on Friday. By the beginning of the fourth week of the program you would be running your target time of 30 minutes on alternate days.

The one-tenth rule provides time for your muscles to recover and adapt to exercise so that you avoid overuse injury. It applies to all forms of exercise, including weight training, where you would increase your weight by one-tenth your target each time you lift weights on alternate days.

4 USE IT OR LOSE IT

The body's capacity to work rises and falls in response to the demands put on its systems. If we're forced to be physically inactive either because of injury, illness or a poor choice of lifestyle, then our bodies respond by reducing their capacities. The muscle cells shrink, losing their power and endurance in a process called atrophy. Bones become thinner and weaker. We become "out of shape." This loss of conditioning can be reversed. If training is interrupted, always restart your activity using the one-tenth rule.

5 FORM FOLLOWS FUNCTION

If we expose the body to the stimulus of exercise followed by a period of recovery, we experience a training response. An appropriate level of exercise followed by an adequate recovery will build strength and endurance by creating cellular changes in your muscles and in your heart and lungs to increase their work capacity. The form or shape of your body changes based on how much training you do. This response is the basis of all improved ability to work or play games that require speed, strength and endurance. But you have to keep it going. Your fitness level is based only on your physical activity during the past 6 weeks. If fitness is not renewed, atrophy follows within weeks.

6 LISTEN TO YOUR BODY

If your body hurts after exercise, pay attention. Pain after exercise shouldn't be ignored. Our bodies can mislead our perception of pain during exercise by producing endorphins, a natural painkiller that often masks overuse injuries. After exercise, the endorphins dissipate and we feel the pain. If the pain begins after weight-bearing or impact activities such as running or aerobic classes that include jumping and landing activity, substitute nonimpact exercise such as cycling or swimming. If the pain persists for more than a day or so, seek medical attention.

7 THE TALK TEST

You know you're working at the right intensity during aerobic activity if you pass the talk test. When running, cycling or doing any aerobic activity, you should be able to carry on a conversation with your partners. If you're breathless or find it uncomfortable to talk, you're too intense in your training. Slow down. Harder effort does not equate with better results! If you were wearing a heart rate monitor, it would show that your pulse rate was out of the aerobic training zone. This could defeat the training effect.

What does it take to burn 600 calories?

HARD INTENSITY ACTIVITY

Hard intensity activity burns 15 to 20 calories every minute. You need 30 to 40 minutes of intense activity to burn 600 calories. Keep it going this long to burn 600 calories:

Practicing martial arts	40 minutes
Cross-country skiing	40 minutes
Playing soccer	40 minutes
Swimming hard	40 minutes
Running moderately	40 minutes
Cycling hard	40 minutes
Rowing hard	40 minutes
Squash	35 minutes
Running hard	30 minutes

POWERFIT HOME STRENGTH PROGRAM

Here's a compact strength-training program that requires no equipment and can be done at home or while traveling. Combine it with the Health-Span 10K Walk Run or the 10K Power Walk program to improve your fitness level. This program should be done on alternate days, about 3 times per week. It increases gradually following the one-tenth rule (page 30).

The PowerFit Home Strength Program includes these exercises:

1 Static V-Sits
2 Eccentric Squats
3 Toe Raise, Heel Drop
4 Push-Ups

The time required for the PowerFit Home Strength Program is about 15 minutes at the outset, increasing to about 30 minutes after 4 weeks. Energy consumption is about 8 to 10 calories per minute.

Here's how you do the exercises.

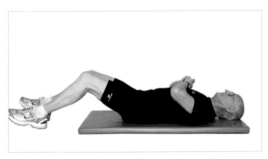

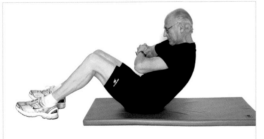

STATIC V-SITS

EXERCISE 1. Static V-Sits

Start by lying on your back with your knees flexed at a 45-degree angle and your feet flat on the floor. Grip your hands together across your chest. Now roll your trunk forward and lift your shoulders off the floor to a 45-degree angle. Keep your feet flat on the floor and your trunk and thighs will form a "V." Hold this position without moving (you're doing a "static" hold).

The target goal for both men and women is to complete 6 repetitions while holding the static V for 20 seconds during each repetition. You'll be able to hold the V-sit for 20 seconds each time if you build up gradually over a 4-week period, using the following schedule:

	DAY 1	DAY 2	DAY 3
WEEK 1	6 times 2 seconds	6 times 4 seconds	6 times 6 seconds
WEEK 2	6 times 8 seconds	6 times 10 seconds	6 times 12 seconds
WEEK 3	6 times 14 seconds	6 times 16 seconds	6 times 18 seconds
WEEK 4	6 times 20 seconds	6 times 20 seconds	6 times 20 seconds

You may find this simple drill difficult at the outset. If you can't get your trunk up to 45 degrees, begin by getting your head up off the carpet without flexing your neck too much. With practice, over several weeks, you'll strengthen your core muscles sufficiently to lift to 45 degrees. If you're having difficulty, modify the program by starting at 1 second and then increasing the time of the "static" hold by 1 second per session. This option would take you 7 weeks to reach the goal.

You may also find the exercise easier if you push your hands together for 10 seconds and then pull them apart for the next 10 seconds during the static hold.

This exercise works wonders for many who suffer from chronic back pain. It strengthens the abdominal muscles that support the back.

EXERCISE 2. *Eccentric Squats*

Start in a standing position with arms extended by your sides. Drop your hips quickly until your thighs are parallel to the floor. The quadriceps muscles in your thighs will contract to stop your fall in what is called an "eccentric" motion. Keeping your feet flat on the floor and your knees over your toes, slowly rise to your original position.

Do 3 sets of repetitions each day, gradually increasing the number of repetitions according to the following schedule:

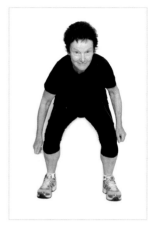

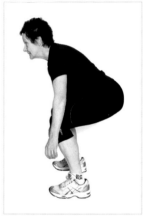

ECCENTRIC SQUATS

	DAY 1	DAY 2	DAY 3
WEEK 1	2 repetitions	4 repetitions	6 repetitions
WEEK 2	8 repetitions	10 repetitions	12 repetitions
WEEK 3	14 repetitions	16 repetitions	18 repetitions
WEEK 4	20 repetitions	20 repetitions	20 repetitions

By the fourth week you'll have reached the goal of 3 sets of 20 repetitions.

This drill helps to stabilize posture by improving strength in the quadriceps and hamstrings of the upper leg. These muscles are vital to limit pain from osteoarthritic conditions of the knee joints.

You can add weights in advanced forms of this drill. Begin with 5 pounds in each hand during the first month, and each month for 3 months increase the weight by 2.5 to 5 pounds. By the fourth month you can be lifting a total of 15 to 20 pounds in each hand for men and 10 to 15 pounds in each hand for women.

Is stretching necessary?

While there is much scientific support for the effectiveness of endurance and strength training in promoting fitness and health, this is not the case for stretching.

In 2004, Shrier published a review report in the *Clinical Journal of Sport Medicine* stating that there is little evidence to prove stretching regimens help to prevent injury. In fact, ballistic stretching or the use of external force by a partner is actually associated with increased risk of injury.

In 2006, Fatouros and his co-researchers at the Democritus University of Thrace reported in the *Journal of Strength and Conditioning Research* the results of a study among men at midlife and older. Study participants completed 10 free-weight exercises while standing and performed them at a moderate intensity 3 times a week for 24 weeks. Even with no stretching exercises, flexibility was improved. This suggests that sport-specific flexibility can be achieved by dynamic loading of the muscle instead of by stretching.

Most injuries are a result of muscle tendon fatigue from overuse, not from inflexibility. When injury occurs, the muscle goes into spasm in an attempt to protect the site, leading to greater inflexibility. Thus the cause lies not in inflexibility but in damage to the muscle tendon. The best therapy is muscle strength retraining, not stretching.

This information does not lessen the value of activities such as yoga and tai chi, which use the weight of the body to train through a full range of motion in a variety of body positions. Nor does this study challenge the universal need for a gradual warm up to increase our core temperature and increase the flexibility of the muscle tendon units before vigorous physical activity.

EXERCISE 3. *Toe Raise, Heel Drop*

Stand on a step or firm raised surface with your forefoot on the step. Rising on one foot at a time, lift your heel up into a toe raise and then drop your heel down so it's below the level of your forefoot. Repeat with the other foot.

Do 3 sets of repetitions each day, gradually increasing the number of repetitions over a period of 4 weeks, as follows:

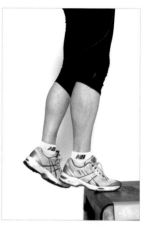

	DAY 1	DAY 2	DAY 3
WEEK 1	2 repetitions	4 repetitions	6 repetitions
WEEK 2	8 repetitions	10 repetitions	12 repetitions
WEEK 3	14 repetitions	16 repetitions	18 repetitions
WEEK 4	20 repetitions	20 repetitions	20 repetitions

By the fourth week you'll have reached the goal of 3 sets of 20 repetitions. This drill maintains flexibility and strength in the lower leg, including the Achilles tendon, and can prevent injury from overuse during running and jumping.

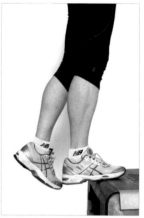

TOE RAISE, HEEL DROP

EXERCISE 4. *Push-Ups*

This classic drill starts with you lying face down on the floor. Your hands should be flat under your shoulders. Now push down and extend your arms while holding your body so that your spine is aligned, with your weight only on your toes.

Do 3 sets of repetitions, gradually increasing the number of repetitions over 4 weeks according to the following schedule:

	DAY 1	DAY 2	DAY 3
WEEK 1	2 repetitions	4 repetitions	6 repetitions
WEEK 2	8 repetitions	10 repetitions	12 repetitions
WEEK 3	14 repetitions	16 repetitions	18 repetitions
WEEK 4	20 repetitions	20 repetitions	20 repetitions

By the fourth week, you'll have reached the goal of 3 sets of 20 repetitions.

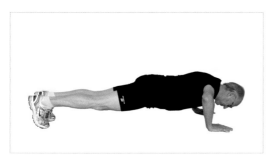

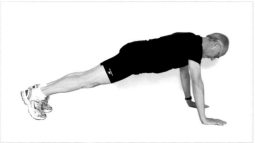

PUSH-UPS

Some may find push-ups hard to do. If so, gradually strengthen your body in 3 stages, as follows:

Phase 1: For the first month, push up against a wall. Stand facing a wall, with feet 3 to 4 feet from the wall. Place your hands on the wall at chest height with your elbows flexed. Extend your arms by pushing away from the wall. Increase the number of repetitions as scheduled above.

Phase 2: During the second month, stand several feet away from a stable table or countertop. Lean forward and place your hands on the surface with your elbows flexed and push up. Increase the number of repetitions as scheduled above.

Phase 3: During the third month, stand at the seat of a stable chair, lean way down and push up. Increase the number of repetitions as scheduled above.

In the fourth month you should be strong enough to begin regular push-ups off the floor.

Push-ups improve strength in the upper body to meet the demands of daily activity and may reduce the risk of tendonitis at the shoulder and elbow.

Combine the PowerFit Home Strength Program with alternate days in the HealthSpan 10K Walk Run or the 10K Power Walk Program to improve your fitness level. Maintaining strength and endurance, along with ideal eating habits, can help you maintain an optimal weight and excellent health.

POWERFIT GYM STRENGTH PROGRAM

This program uses a weight training facility or gymnasium, and can be modified to include the specific equipment available. Combined with the HealthSpan 10K Walk Run or the 10K Power Walk Program, this Power-Fit Gym Strength Program can provide the fitness you need with just 2 basic components. Do these exercises on alternate days, about 3 times per week. Each session should be followed the next day with aerobic or recovery work. This program increases gradually following the one-tenth rule (page 30).

The PowerFit Gym Strength Program includes 2 basic components.

1 Using Stationary Weight Training Machines, 1 set of 8 repetitions of each of the following:

» Shoulder press
» Overhead press
» Bent-over rowing
» Crunch
» Pull-downs
» Leg press

2 In Circuit Training, 3 sets of varied repetitions of each of the following:

» Step-Ups
» Biceps Curls
» Eccentric Squats
» Toe Raise, Heel Drop
» Static V-Sits

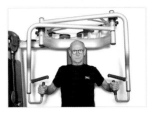

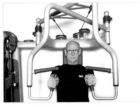

SHOULDER PRESS

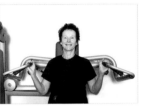

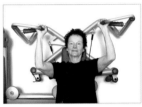

OVERHEAD PRESS

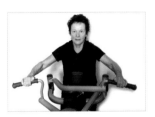

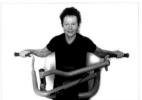

BENT-OVER ROWING

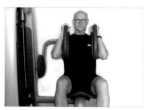

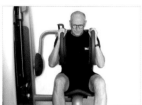

CRUNCH

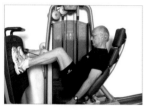

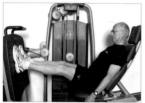

LEG PRESS

The time required for the PowerFit Gym Strength Program is about 15 to 20 minutes at the outset, increasing to about 30 minutes after 24 weeks. Energy consumption is about 10 calories per minute.

Here's what to do.

Stationary Weight Training Machines The selection of machines available in each gym will vary. Adapt the list of exercises provided here to the equipment available. The goal is to develop maximal strength with only 1 set of exercises of just 8 repetitions at each machine station. Start with a weight that provides a challenge only on the last 2 repetitions. You can never be wrong with starting with a modest weight and gradually building up over time. Since you're doing only 1 set of 8 reps, choose a weight that's easy in the first 6 reps but becomes more difficult in the last 2 reps. Move to the next machine after completing 8 reps. Increase the weight you choose if the last 2 reps become too easy after several weeks. When you've completed the single set of 8 reps at each machine, move on to the circuit training.

Circuit Training In circuit training we do 5 exercises, each one followed immediately by the next, until all 5 drills have been completed. Repeat the circuit 2 more times for a total of 3 sets. The goal is to gradually increase the weight resistance each month until you reach the target. If you follow the schedule for gradually increasing weight and repetitions per set, by the fourth week you'll have reached your target number of repetitions. Keep it going and by the fourth month you'll have reached your target.

EQUIPMENT NEEDED
» Stable gym step that is about 10 inch (25 cm) high
» Dumbbell weights ranging from 3 to 5 lb to 12 to 15 lb for women, and 20 lb for men
» Athletic shoes

EXERCISE 1. *Step-Ups*

This exercise improves strength and cardiovascular endurance. Stand in front of a gym step, with dumbbell weights in each hand and arms extended by your sides. Step up onto the gym step and then step down. Alternate lead legs. Begin with 3 to 5 lb dumbbell weights and increase the amount of weight each month.

The target goal for women is to carry 12 to 15 lb in each hand while stepping 20 times during each of 3 sets.

The target goal for men is to carry 20 lb in each hand while stepping 20 times during each of 3 sets.

Gradually increase the weight carried according to the following schedule:

FIRST MONTH	3 to 5 lb
SECOND MONTH	5 to 10 lb
THIRD MONTH	10 to 15 lb
FOURTH MONTH	15 to 20 lb

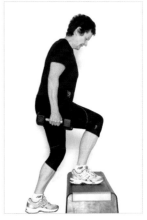

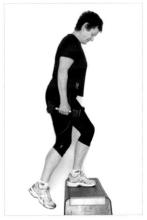

STEP-UPS

And gradually increase the number of repetitions:

	DAY 1	DAY 2	DAY 3
WEEK 1	2 repetitions	4 repetitions	6 repetitions
WEEK 2	8 repetitions	10 repetitions	12 repetitions
WEEK 3	14 repetitions	16 repetitions	18 repetitions
WEEK 4	20 repetitions	20 repetitions	20 repetitions

This exercise strengthens the quadriceps and hamstrings in your upper leg as well as the gastrocnemius (the muscle at the back of the lower calf). All are essential in walking and stair climbing.

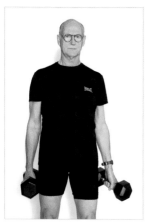

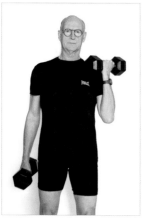

BICEPS CURL

EXERCISE 2. *Biceps Curl*

Start in a standing position with dumbbells in each hand and arms extended by your sides. Bend both elbows and raise the weights to your shoulders. Slowly lower the weights to their original position.

The target goal for women is to lift and lower 12 to 15 lb in each hand 20 times during each of 3 sets.

The target goal for men is to lift and lower 20 lb in each hand 20 times during each of 3 sets.

Gradually increase the weight carried according to the following schedule:

FIRST MONTH	3 to 5 lb
SECOND MONTH	5 to 10 lb
THIRD MONTH	10 to 15 lb
FOURTH MONTH	15 to 20 lb

And gradually increase the number of repetitions:

	DAY 1	DAY 2	DAY 3
WEEK 1	2 repetitions	4 repetitions	6 repetitions
WEEK 2	8 repetitions	10 repetitions	12 repetitions
WEEK 3	14 repetitions	16 repetitions	18 repetitions
WEEK 4	20 repetitions	20 repetitions	20 repetitions

This drill improves strength in the biceps and triceps muscles of the upper arm, which are essential for all household tasks. Strength in these muscles may reduce the risk of tennis elbow.

EXERCISE 3. *Eccentric Squats*

Start in a standing position with dumbbells in each hand and arms extended by your sides. Drop your hips quickly until your thighs are parallel to the floor. The quadriceps muscles in your thighs will contract to stop your fall in what is called an "eccentric" motion. Keeping your feet flat on the floor and your knees over your toes, slowly rise to your original position.

The target goal for women is to carry 12 to 15 lb in each hand while squatting 20 times during each of 3 sets. The target goal for men is to carry 20 lb in each hand while squatting 20 times during each of 3 sets.

Gradually increase the weight carried according to the following schedule:

FIRST MONTH	3 to 5 lb
SECOND MONTH	5 to 10 lb
THIRD MONTH	10 to 15 lb
FOURTH MONTH	15 to 20 lb

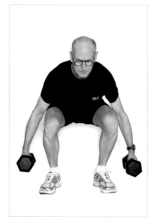

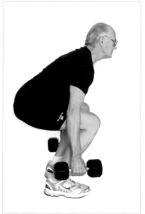

ECCENTRIC SQUATS

And gradually increase the number of repetitions:

	DAY 1	DAY 2	DAY 3
WEEK 1	2 repetitions	4 repetitions	6 repetitions
WEEK 2	8 repetitions	10 repetitions	12 repetitions
WEEK 3	14 repetitions	16 repetitions	18 repetitions
WEEK 4	20 repetitions	20 repetitions	20 repetitions

This drill helps to stabilize posture by improving strength in the quadriceps and hamstrings of the upper leg. These muscles are vital to limit pain from osteoarthritic conditions of the knee joints.

EXERCISE 4. *Toe Raise, Heel Drop*

Stand on a step or firm raised surface with your forefoot on the step. Lifting one foot at a time, lift your heel up into a toe raise and then drop your heel down so it is below the level of your forefoot. Repeat with the other foot.

The target goal for both men and women is to raise and lower each heel 20 times during each of 3 sets of repetitions. Increase the number of repetitions of a period of 4 weeks, as follows:

	DAY 1	DAY 2	DAY 3
WEEK 1	2 repetitions	4 repetitions	6 repetitions
WEEK 2	8 repetitions	10 repetitions	12 repetitions
WEEK 3	14 repetitions	16 repetitions	18 repetitions
WEEK 4	20 repetitions	20 repetitions	20 repetitions

This drill maintains flexibility and strength in the lower leg, including the Achilles tendon, and can prevent injury from overuse during running and jumping.

EXERCISE 5. *Static V-Sits*

Start by lying on your back with your knees flexed at a 45-degree angle and your feet flat on the floor. Grip your hands together across your chest. Now roll your trunk forward and lift your shoulders off the floor to a 45-degree angle. Keep your feet flat on the floor and your trunk and thighs will form a "V." Hold this position without moving in a static hold.

The target goal for both men and women is to complete 6 repetitions while holding the static V for 20 seconds during each repetition. You'll be able to hold for 20 seconds each time if you build up gradually over a 4-week period.

Gradually increase the length of time you hold the V-sit according to this schedule:

	DAY 1	DAY 2	DAY 3
WEEK 1	6 times 2 seconds	6 times 4 seconds	6 times 6 seconds
WEEK 2	6 times 8 seconds	6 times 10 seconds	6 times 12 seconds
WEEK 3	6 times 14 seconds	6 times 16 seconds	6 times 18 seconds
WEEK 4	6 times 20 seconds	6 times 20 seconds	6 times 20 seconds

You may find this simple drill difficult at the outset. If you can't get your trunk up to 45 degrees, begin by getting your head up off the carpet without flexing your neck too much. With practice, over several weeks, you'll strengthen your core muscles sufficiently to reach the target goal. If you're having difficulty, modify the program by starting at 1 second and increasing the time of the "static" hold by 1 second per session. This would take 7 weeks to reach the goal. You may also find the exercise easier if you push your hands together for 10 seconds and then pull them apart for the next 10 seconds during the static hold.

This exercise works wonders for many who suffer from chronic back pain. It strengthens the abdominal muscles that support the back.

Remember that when you've completed the 5 exercises in sequence, you need to repeat 2 more circuits for a total of 3 sets of the 5 exercises each session. Once you reach the target goal for each exercise, maintain the schedule during the following weeks for overall strength and fitness.

Exercise programs are like food—they come in all colors and tastes. There's no single exercise program that's the only approach. All physical activity training for us in midlife or beyond is aimed at maintaining the strength and endurance we need to engage easily in everyday tasks throughout our lives.

In the straight stretch: Setting realistic goals

Your Start Fresh goals are clear:
» Improve your HealthSpan report card.
» Review your lifestyle.
» Choose an activity that suits your body type.
» Choose physical activities that spark your interest and passion and fit into your work and family responsibilities.
» Choose multiple forms of activities that burn a total of 600 calories per day.

The Chef and Doctor's Personal Exercise Prescription

Diane and I try to be physically active 5 to 6 days per week. We try to mix a pattern of 1 day of intense exercise with 1 day of moderate intensity or rest. For example: Monday, Wednesday and Friday, our workload could be heavy, but on Tuesday, Thursday and the weekend days, we recover or rest. This plan is entirely flexible and is modified frequently to match a busy schedule of other activities.

Our days of intense activity include 1 hour in the gym doing the following:

AEROBIC COMPONENT

We work for 30 minutes at a pulse rate of 70% to 85% of maximum for a total energy output of 300 calories.

EXERCISE 1. Stationary Bicycle
» duration: 10 minutes
» revolutions per minute (rpm): 90 to 100
» pulse rate: 70% of maximum (105 beats per minute)
» energy output: 100 calories

EXERCISE 2. Concept II Rowing Ergometer
» duration: 10 minutes
» strokes per minute: 28
» pace: 2 minutes 8.5 seconds per 500 meters
» distance: 1.25 miles (2,000 meters)
» pulse rate: 85% of maximum (127 beats per minute)
» energy output: 100 calories

EXERCISE 3. Treadmill Walking
» duration: 10 minutes
» speed: 4.5 miles (7.25 kilometers) per hour
» grade: 4.5%
» pulse rate: 75% of maximum (112 beats per minute)
» energy output: 100 calories

STRENGTH COMPONENT

We work for 30 minutes at a pulse rate of 70% to 80% of maximum for a total energy output of 300 calories.

EXERCISE 1. *Stationary Weight Training Machines*

1 set of 8 repetitions at maximal weight of each of the following:

» shoulder press
» overhead press
» bent-over rowing
» crunch
» pull-downs
» leg press

EXERCISE 2. *Circuit Training*

While I hold 20 lb in each hand and Diane holds 15 lb in each hand, we do 3 sets of 20 repetitions of each of the following:

» step-ups
» squats
» biceps curls
» toe raises, heel drops

EXERCISE 3. *Static V-Sits*

» 6 sets of 20-second static holds

The following day of recovery generally involves walking, hiking, snowshoeing or cycling. During these exercises our pulse rates will be at 60% to 65% of maximum or lower. We try to obtain 60 to 120 minutes of these more moderate forms of exercise in order to meet our target of burning 600 calories every day.

These targets are modified to synchronize with other time commitments. For example, if we're traveling or miss some period of time in the gymnasium for other reasons, on our return we lower the intensity using the one-tenth rule (page 30). We gradually build the intensity back up over 3 or 4 weeks.

"TELL ME
WHAT YOU EAT
AND I WILL
TELL YOU
WHAT YOU ARE."

–Jean-Anthelme Brillat-Savarin, 1826

fuel to keep going!

THE CHEF TELLS YOU HOW TO EAT RIGHT

The war on the waist won't be won by sweat equity alone. You need to combine fitness with healthy eating in order to reach your ideal waist measurement. Only a combination of proper food choices and exercise will help you succeed. Good food choices are especially important at midlife when metabolism slows and often our food intake increases. No one told us in our youth that we'd have to switch to half-rations in our fifth decade.

The solution: Eating right for life

The best way to eat right to maintain good health at midlife and beyond is to follow these 7 steps to eat right for life:

1 Forget diets; they don't work. Why do we gain weight? It all comes down to calories. It's eating too much and not exercising that makes us fat. It's intake equals output. Managing your weight and your health is not only something we should do all the time, but something that's easy to do when it becomes a lifetime commitment instead of a temporary crash diet.

2 Use self-control. Avoid the "eat everything" diet, where you promise to lose it tomorrow. If you're overindulging, cut down on your portions. Eat 20% to 30% less food at each meal. Serve meals on a salad or breakfast plate instead of a dinner plate; unless you're a high-level athlete, this really will be enough food for you. It's a simple permanent change that will make a long-term difference to your weight.

3 "Under-size" me. Portions of meat, poultry and fish should be the size of the palm of your hand or the size of a deck of cards. Fruits and vegetables should be the star attraction, with five to eight ½-cup (125 mL) servings daily. Add zing to your dishes by adding exotic spices and fresh herbs without adding calories.

4 Finish each meal when you're 80% full. Never fill your stomach; always leave some room. Take a break halfway through anything you eat to check if you're actually still hungry. Most of the time we keep eating because food is available rather than because we're hungry.

5 Eat slowly. It takes your brain 10 to 15 minutes to realize that you've eaten. If you eat quickly, by the time your brain signals that your stomach is full you'll have eaten almost twice the amount of food that you need.

6 Water and veggies fill you up. Serve water with every meal to help fill you up. Start every meal with a fresh salad. The variety of greens available today is staggering: from the classic iceberg, romaine and red leaf lettuce or spinach, to the exotic ruffled leaves of curly endive. Use your imagination by adding color and flavor with local tomatoes, peppers, cucumbers and other produce.

7 Do we really need to snack between meals? If you're genuinely hungry, then reach for fresh fruit. Snacking on chips, chocolate bars or cookies adds unwanted calories. If stress or lack of sleep make you reach for carbs, go for a healthy carb such as strawberries or a banana, rather than a candy bar or chocolate chip cookies. Get berry calm.

The chef and doctor in the kitchen: Stocking up
An important key to eating well begins by stocking your pantry, refrigerator and freezer with healthy foods.

THE PANTRY

Chocolate, chocolate, chocolate: A nibble a day of dark chocolate helps lower blood pressure without packing on the pounds. Chocolate with 62% to 72% cacao offers heart protective benefits, but researchers have worried that the added sugar, fat and calories would cancel out any good the chocolate might do. Now it seems just a 30-calorie bite of dark chocolate—equivalent to 6.8 grams or ¼ oz—can lower blood pressure without weight gain or other negative side effects. Hurray!

Oils: Oil, like all fat, should be used sparingly. For sautéing meats and vegetables, use polyunsaturated oils such as safflower, sunflower, grape seed or canola, or pure olive oil (a monounsaturated oil). Select a good quality extra virgin olive oil (from the first pressing of the olives) for your salads.

Vinegars: Balsamic vinegar from Modena, Italy, is perfect for salad dressings such as Basic Balsamic Vinaigrette (page 103). I also like to vary the vinegars, from sherry, champagne, white and red wines to citrus fruits.

Fast food:
Slow burn

Did you know that if you decided to tackle a Big Mac, French fries and a large milkshake for lunch, you would consume 2,200 calories? You would then have to walk almost a marathon (22 miles or 35 kilometers) to burn the energy provided. If you didn't walk, then the 2,200 calories could be converted to 0.63 pounds of body fat. Does "super size" mean my weight? I think so!

Take a daily multivitamin

As a form of insurance, Diane and I take a simple, low-cost multivitamin and mineral supplementation daily to insure that we have an adequate amount of these trace substances. Women with low caloric intake are prone to develop iron deficiency anemia as well as a calcium deficiency related osteoporosis. It may be unnecessary to supplement vitamins and minerals but the use of supplements may have a place when caloric restriction or food allergies are present.

The happy spices: Grind your own spices from around the world to add flavor to your favorite foods. Experiment and enjoy. But keep spices away from the stove, where they quickly lose their flavor, and use them within 6 months of purchase.

Salt and pepper: Use salt sparingly, just to season lightly to reduce water retention and weight gain and to reduce blood pressure. Maldon salt, from the English coast, is a popular choice for many chefs. Or try red salt from Hawaii or *fleur de sel* from France. My choice of pepper is a blend of 4 different peppercorns (black, green, white and pink) with whole allspice. Or try Tellicherry peppercorns from the southwest coast of India, the finest pepper in the world.

Condiments: How many sauces, chutneys, mustards, pickles and relishes do you have in your kitchen? I have dozens. Some stars include Hellmann's light mayonnaise, which is the only mayonnaise I use and a favorite with restaurant chefs. You should also include Dijon mustard, chutneys and tapenades.

Grains: Stock your pantry with whole grain pastas, bulgur wheat, couscous, brown rice, arborio rice, polenta and quinoa.

Go nuts: Roasted nuts and peanut butter are, mmm, good. A little goes a long way, though, so don't over indulge: 2 Tbsp (30 mL) of peanut butter provides nearly 200 calories.

Red wine: A perfect complement to any meal, a 5 oz (150 mL) glass of red a day keeps our body rhythms flowing, weighing in at 200 calories. Women should limit their alcohol intake to 1 glass a day.

Green tea: So soothing, green tea is also full of healthy antioxidants.

Coffee: Enjoy but limit your intake to 1 or 2 cups a day to reduce your caffeine intake.

THE REFRIGERATOR
Think Fresh. Buy Fresh. Eat Fresh.

Fresh fruits and vegetables: Shop on the weekends to stock your refrigerator and fruit bowls with locally grown organic fruits and veggies whenever possible because they're grown without harmful pesticides. Replenish your fresh foods midweek. Home delivery of fresh local farm produce has become a popular alternative. Consider ordering a bin of organic vegetables to be delivered to your home each week. Always have a supply of the following fruits and veggies on hand: tomatoes (Italians say never put tomatoes in the refrigerator because they lose flavor and become pulpy), onions, potatoes, yams and bananas. Also stock up on prewashed greens, lemons, limes and fruit that's in season.

Organic eggs and meat: Certified organic farms create a smaller carbon footprint than conventional farms, and animals that produce organic meat, poultry, eggs and dairy products don't take antibiotics or growth hormones that can damage your health.

Dairy: Always have on hand low-fat yogurt, low-fat cottage cheese and skim milk.

Juices: Pure fruit and vegetable juices contribute to your daily intake of 5 to 8 fruits and vegetables but remember that besides being rich in some vitamins and minerals they add to your total caloric intake. Moderation rules!

THE FREEZER
Be Prepared.

Shop at warehouse stores to buy frozen food in bulk packages. When you get home, divide them into smaller 2 cup (500 mL) packages, enough to serve 2 people. Maintain a supply of frozen Asian vegetables to use in stir frying, frozen fruits for fruit smoothies, chicken breasts, peppered smoked salmon, corn and whole wheat flour tortillas, pita bread and low-fat pizzas. Prepare Start Fresh recipes that freeze well so you always have a meal on hand when you're short of time (see sidebar on page 53).

How to make weekday meals easy, tasty and healthy

With your kitchen stocked with healthy ingredients, you'll be more motivated to prepare dinner after a hectic day at work. To make it even easier, make a 4-day menu plan based on easy, quick, no-fuss recipes such as those in this book. Read through the recipe section and find the recipes you'd like to prepare. Read them thoroughly and prepare a grocery list, categorizing the necessary items as refrigerator foods, frozen foods or pantry staples so you don't have to repeat trips down the grocery aisles. Then do the shopping on the weekend when you have more time. When you have a supply of delicious food waiting for you at home, you won't panic at the end of the workday and resort to fast food takeout.

When cooking at home, big-batch it! Prepare 1 or 2 extra meals during the weekend and plan for 1 meal out, leaving only 2 or 3 weeknights for live cooking. Prepare double portions and freeze the rest. Double-batch the Grilled Lemon Chicken with Red Pepper Chutney (page 171) to freeze and pull out for lunch sandwiches. Also double-batch rice so you have one batch to freeze to serve with Asian stir-fried vegetables, meat or seafood.

Start prepping the recipe the night before. Cut the vegetables, make the dressing and marinate the meat. It will make life easier when you arrive home to prepare dinner.

Post the recipes to remind you what has to be pulled out of the freezer for the next night's dinner.

If you really have no time to cook, rely on your local markets, family delis and catering establishments that offer an international selection of healthy take-out foods, from homemade pasta sauces to rotisserie chicken and meats, salads, soups, sandwiches and vegetables. They're made daily and are generally free from preservatives and salt.

MONDAY-TO-FRIDAY MENU PLANNING

With busy commitments during the week, I don't have time to spend preparing fussy lunches or dinners every day. Here's a taste of how Doug and I eat during the week while on the run.

Breakfast We usually start our day with Doug's skim-milk lattes, a glass of 100% pure fruit juice (our favorite is Ocean Spray unsweetened pure cranberry juice) and vitamins (see sidebar on page 50) before our workout.

After our workout and before noon Tea and one of the following:
» The Fitness Group Smoothie (page 61) or Suzie's Wake-Up Jumpstart (page 60).

- » 1 slice whole wheat toast or bagel with peanut butter and Nutella Hazelnut Spread, or 1 of Jen's Power Muffins (page 65) or 2 small Max's Branberry Muffins (page 64).
- » Porridge (not instant) with sliced bananas or blueberries, warmed skim milk and 1 Tbsp (15 mL) maple syrup.
- » Coco's Fruit, Granola and Yogurt Parfait (page 62) with 1 slice of wholewheat or fruit and nut toast or 1 whole wheat bagel, a little peanut butter and Nutella Hazelnut Spread.

Sandwiches   We share a sandwich, plus a small side salad or 1 cup (250 mL) of soup each, such as Gazpacho (page 81), Carrot Tomato Soup (page 79) or a heart-smart commercial soup, and 1 piece of fruit.

Salads   If I make a salad—such as Jane's Grilled Tuna Salad with Mango Pineapple Salsa (page 93), Tomato, Red Onion and White Bean Salad (page 83), Asian Noodle Salad (page 97) or Diane's Westcoaster Salad with Maple Balsamic Vinaigrette (page 99)—I add 3 or 4 whole wheat crackers or 1 or 2 slices of sourdough whole wheat country bread minus the butter, and 1 piece of fruit.

Dinner choices   During the week, we usually enjoy the menus I've suggested for weekday dinners. I also rely on the frozen dishes that I've tucked in the freezer (see sidebar). We enjoy the many healthy fresh take-out choices that our grocery markets and delis offer to spoil us when we simply don't have time to cook.

Evening pick-me-up   Usually 1 piece of fruit satisfies our sweet tooth, and a little wedge of dark chocolate to tease the palate.

MENUS FOR WEEKDAY DINNERS

Planning weekday dinners is always a dilemma. But follow the guidelines (page 52) and life will be more relaxed when preparing dinners after working all day. Here are a few of our most requested weekday family dinners.

Mexican Night

- » Arugula and Black Olive Salad (page 95) or Avocado and Peppers Salad (page 91)
- » Santa Fe Corn Pie (page 74) or Chicken Tortilla Pie (page 173)
- » Guacamole (page 135) with corn chips
- » fresh pineapple and kiwi

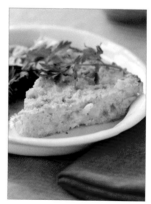

SANTA FE CORN PIE

Hearty Fare

» tossed green salad with peppers, cucumber, green onions and tomatoes
» Basic Balsamic Vinaigrette (page 103)
» Vegetarian Chili (page 156)
» Champion Cornbread (page 158) or wholegrain bread
» Lucia's Banana Ice with Berry Purée (page 185)

Westcoast Salad Night

» Carrot Tomato Soup (page 79) or low-fat deli soup
» Diane's Westcoaster Salad with Maple Balsamic Vinaigrette (page 99)
» wholegrain or sourdough bread
» fresh fruit platter and frozen yogurt

Weekend entertaining

Weekends are the time for all of us to let loose in the kitchen to prepare family favorites and try new recipes. The recipes in this book include some of the most requested signature dishes from my *Chef on the Run* series of cookbooks, but with a major difference. I've reduced the total caloric content by choosing low-fat ingredients to meet our criteria for healthy eating. At the same time, I was determined not to sacrifice taste and flavor. My new recipes have also taken time and patience to create—tantalizing dishes from around the world that we can all enjoy within our caloric needs. What was the reaction from the tasting judges of friends and family? Their final answer: "Wow, Diane, we're savoring every bite."

MENUS FOR WEEKEND ENTERTAINING

It's a special treat to be invited to someone's home for food, fun and entertainment. Weekends are the best time to entertain, either for brunch or for an evening dinner party. We don't need a special occasion to give us the incentive to invite family and friends over to enjoy good food and lively conversation, and a meal doesn't have to blow your month's budget either!

Here are 5 menu ideas using various recipes in this book, something for every occasion. The key to all the recipes in *Start Fresh!*, whether for entertaining or for every day, is that they meet our caloric balance and at the same time make our taste buds tingle! Create your own menus to suit your time and number of guests. Remember, take advantage of your favorite deli, bakery or specialty shop to make entertaining easier if time runs out.

Your local wine merchant would be happy to recommend wines to complement your specific menu.

Tex-Mex Salmon Taco Party

Mexican cuisine spells "informal dining" enjoyed by all ages. Pick up the ingredients from a Mexican deli or your local supermarket, including the salsas and guacamole if rushed. Start off with a chilled bottle of Mexican beer (don't forget the lime) or a glass of Crangria Blanca (page 116) and let the party begin!

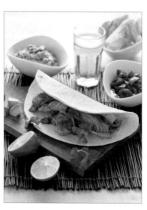

TEX-MEX SALMON TACOS

» Mexican beer
» Crangria Blanca (page 116)
» Tex-Mex Salmon Tacos (page 177) and/or Tequila Chicken (page 174) or Chicken Tortilla Pie (page 173)
» Speedy Refried Beans (page 154)
» Guacamole (page 135)
» Tomato and Red Onion Salsa (page 110)
» Mango Pineapple Salsa (page 111)
» corn chips
» whole wheat tortillas
» Lime Mousse with Tropical Fruit (page 181) or Aztec Ice Cream with Lime Sauce (page 186)

Doug's July Birthday Celebration: Spanish Cava and Tapas

Since we're almost guaranteed a warm, balmy day to celebrate Doug's birthday, which is in July, I usually plan a cold make-ahead menu. If you want to do something similar, try this menu. Start off with a bubbly to go with the Spanish tapas dishes, or offer a selection of Spanish wines. Follow up with the spectacular Cobb Salad St. Tropez, and a classic almond tart for dessert. Let everyone help themselves.

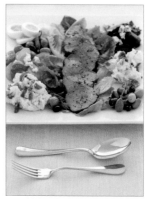

COBB SALAD ST. TROPEZ

» Roasted Almonds with Smoked Paprika (page 126)
» Artichoke Frittata (page 121)
» Feta Cheese with Lemon Zest, Pine Nuts and Olives (page 128)
» Kasbar Duck Confit (page 125)
» flatbreads and whole wheat crackers
» Cobb Salad St. Tropez (page 85)
» Spanish Almond Tart with Orange and Date Compote (page 183)
» orange sorbet

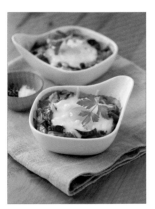

EGGS WITH QUICK
RATATOUILLE

Santa Fe Brunch

On a visit to Santa Fe, New Mexico, Doug and I had the most scrumptious Huevos Rancheros we have ever eaten, with braised pork and a spicy tomato sauce. I've worked on this recipe (page 70) over the years and I think I've come pretty close to the original dish. The sauce takes a little time to prepare, but can be made 1 to 2 days ahead, or frozen. When running out of time, whip up Eggs with Quick Ratatouille (page 69). It also gets rave reviews.

» Champagne and orange juice
» Vincent's Huevos Rancheros with Braised Pork and Spicy Tomato Sauce (page 70) or Eggs with Quick Ratatouille (page 69)
» Avocado and Peppers Salad (page 91)
» Santa Fe Corn Pie (page 74)
» whole wheat flour tortillas
» corn chips
» pineapple and kiwi fruit plate
» pineapple and mango sorbets

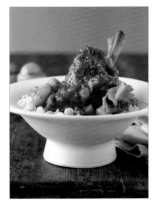

LAMB TAGINE WITH
GLAZED CINNAMON FIGS

Taste of Morocco

One of the most memorable trips for Doug and me was our 3-week sojourn to Morocco. Experiencing their vibrant healthy cuisine was unforgettable: from the simple Atlas Mountains Berber villages' fresh eggs and flatbreads, to the Sahara Desert banquet and the Moroccan chefs' specialties served at our *riad* (hotel). This menu reflects the fragrant flavors of Moroccan cooking. Most of the menu can be prepared ahead of time.

» Roasted Red Pepper Hummus (page 120)
» Mushrooms with Garlic (page 127)
» Kasbar Duck Confit (page 125)
» Rand's Roasted Beets with Yogurt (page 130)
» Pita Crisps (page 159) and flatbreads
» Lamb Tagine with Glazed Cinnamon Figs (page 165)
» Couscous with Chickpeas (page 148)
» Moroccan Melon and Ginger Fruit Salad (page 102)
» Spanish Almond Tart with Orange and Date Compote (page 183)
» Mint Tea (page 115)

Asian Express

Beijing, Shanghai and Singapore were the highlights of a trip we made to Asia in 2001. This menu represents the many dishes we enjoyed as we toured these magnificent cities.

> » Maui Sweet Onion Soup with Sun-Dried
>   Tomato Chèvre Crostini (page 77)
> » rice crackers
> » Chicken Satay with Spicy Peanut Dip (page 136)
> » China Grill Vegetable Rice (page 155)
> » Lime Mousse with Tropical Fruit (page 181)
>   or Jill's Berries in Rosé Wine Jelly (page 187)
> » green tea
> » fortune cookies

THE RECIPES

It was an exciting challenge for me to select about 40 signature dishes from almost 3 decades of the *Chef on the Run* cookbooks and to rework them to meet our healthier mandate, which features vegetables, fruits and whole grains and limits foods high in saturated fats. I had to modify recipes to reduce saturated fats, sodium intake and total calories without sacrificing taste and visual appeal. That meant I had my work in the kitchen cut out for me.

The first step was to not buy butter, replacing it with olive or vegetable oil for cooking and throwing away the butter dish for breads. If you do the same, I think you'll discover you don't miss it. The next step was to replace the salt shaker with freshly chopped herbs and a sprinkle of freshly ground pepper. I then substituted whole wheat grains for white flour and substituted low-fat dairy products for whipping cream and sour cream. The reward: recipes that help you maintain a healthy weight (the proof is on the scales) and feel more energetic. What could be a more positive balance?

Eating is one of life's most pleasurable essentials, and there's nothing more satisfying than a home-cooked meal prepared especially for you, whether it's a simple weekday meal or a special Sunday dinner. But would my healthy recipes win over the tasting team?

"Fresh, innovative, stylish and delicious" was the feedback I received from my tasting enthusiasts. They all agreed that both the signature and new recipes do indeed entice, seduce and bring pleasure. Tasters especially loved the new recipes that I have developed from our recent travels to Asia, Spain, Morocco, Hawaii and the Caribbean. I hope you'll have as much fun cooking these healthy recipes as I had creating them.

Per serving analysis

To ensure that the recipes also meet our health criteria, we evaluated the ingredients using the nutritional analysis available at www.caloriesper-hour.com. A per-serving analysis accompanies each recipe and shows the total calories per serving as well as grams of carbohydrate, fiber, fat and protein and milligrams of sodium.

The recommended daily intake balances: 52% carbohydrates, 33% fats and 15% proteins. Total sodium intake should be less than 1,500 milligrams per day. Fiber intake should be at least 18 milligrams daily. Use the per-serving nutritional analysis for each recipe to watch that your daily intake of these nutrients stays within recommended daily values.

Walk off those calories

FAST FOOD	CALORIE INTAKE	FAT CONSUMED	DISTANCE YOU NEED TO WALK
Big Mac sandwich	530 calories	29 grams	5.3 miles / 8.5 km
french fries	570 calories	30 grams	5.7 miles / 9.2 km
large chocolate triple thick shake	1,600 calories	27 grams	16 miles / 26 km
mocha frappuccino vente	500 calories	17 grams	5 miles / 8 km
chocolate chip plain muffin	430 calories	14 grams	4.3 miles / 7 km
chocolate cream–filled doughnut	350 calories	20 grams	3.5 miles / 5.6 km
Hawaiian Feast large pizza, 4 slices	520 calories	32 grams	5.2 miles / 8.4 km
chocolate chip cookie dough ice cream, double scoop	620 calories	40 grams	6.2 miles / 10K
chocolate fudge brownie low-fat frozen yogurt, double scoop	400 calories	5 grams	4 miles / 6.4 km
chocolate low-fat sorbet, double scoop	260 calories	1 gram	2.6 miles / 4.2 km

Choices really do matter! Choosing a double scoop of sorbet (260 calories) instead of a double scoop of ice cream (620 calories) saves you 3.6 miles (5.8 km) of walking. Choosing calorie-free green tea instead of a muffin and a frappuccino at coffee break saves you a 2½-hour walk over 9.3 miles (15 km) to burn those calories. The take-home message? Intelligent food choices are just as important as exercise to start fresh and stay healthy.

off the blocks

Breakfasts and Brunches to Start the Day Right

SUZIE'S WAKE-UP JUMPSTART

Makes 1 drink, about 1½ cups (375 mL)

PER SERVING
276 calories
4 g protein
1 g fat
63 g carbohydrate
4 g fiber
24 mg sodium

When Jennifer and I opened Tomato Fresh Food Café we tasted dozens of fruit combinations for our fresh juice bar. We named this combination "The Suzie Q," after my daughter-in-law, Suzanne. It became Tomato's bestselling fruit smoothie. This is an updated version that uses tropical fruit. It's totally refreshing and filling. Substitute strawberries for the mangoes and peaches, if you prefer.

1 cup (250 mL) orange juice

½ cup (125 mL) peeled and sliced mangoes or peaches (or combination), fresh or frozen

½ ripe banana, peeled and sliced into chunks

2 Tbsp (30 mL) low-fat vanilla or tropical yogurt

2 or 3 ice cubes (if using fresh, not frozen fruit)

Toss everything into the jar of a blender. If using fresh fruit, add the ice cubes. Blend well. Now you're ready to start your day!

THE FITNESS GROUP SMOOTHIE

Barbara Crompton opened The Fitness Group in Vancouver in the early 1980s. Barbara's fitness classes were jammed and she led the way for the thousands of fitness trainers across North America who are changing our lives for the better. After Barbara put us through our paces, we all lined up for her famous smoothie. The original recipe added honey, but it's sweet enough and more calorie friendly with fruit alone. It's the perfect start to your day, every day!

1 cup (250 mL) fresh or frozen strawberries or other fruits

1 ripe banana

½ cup (125 mL) skim milk

½ cup (125 mL) low-fat vanilla yogurt

1 Tbsp (15 mL) wheat germ

2 or 3 ice cubes (if using fresh, not frozen fruit)

Throw the strawberries, banana, skim milk, yogurt and wheat germ into the jar of a blender. Add the ice cubes if using fresh fruit and blend at high speed for a few seconds. Enjoy!

Makes 1 drink, about 2 cups (500 mL)

PER SERVING
280 calories
14 g protein
1 g fat
54 g carbohydrate
6 g fiber
140 mg sodium

Chef's Secret

WHEAT GERM Adding wheat germ instead of the original wheat bran really boosts our vital nutrients such as B vitamins plus potassium, phosphorus, calcium, zinc and magnesium. Store wheat germ in the refrigerator, as wheat germ oil degrades quickly when exposed to extremes in temperature, oxidization and light.

COCO'S FRUIT, GRANOLA *and* YOGURT PARFAIT

Serves 1

....

PER SERVING
221 calories
12 g protein
3 g fat
39 g carbohydrate
3 g fiber
318 mg sodium

Chef's Secret

REACH FOR THE OJ For a pick-me-up during the day, it's nutritionally better to drink ½ cup (125 mL) 100% pure and natural orange or other pure fruit juice rather than 2 cups (500 mL) sugar-laden soft drinks. Orange juice contains vitamin C and is only 56 calories while the soft drink contains 194 calories and no nutrients.

Our granddaughter Coco loves this healthy breakfast treat and it's Doug and my favorite morning pick-me-up after a workout.

½ cup (125 mL) mixed fresh fruit

....

¼ cup (60 mL) low-fat granola plus a sprinkle for garnish

....

¼ cup (60 mL) low-fat yogurt

....

¼ cup (60 mL) low-fat cottage cheese (optional)

Spread half the fruit on the bottom of a dessert bowl, and then layer half of the amounts of granola, yogurt and cottage cheese (if using). Repeat the layers with the remaining half of the fruit, granola, yogurt and cottage cheese (if using), ending with a sprinkle of granola on top.

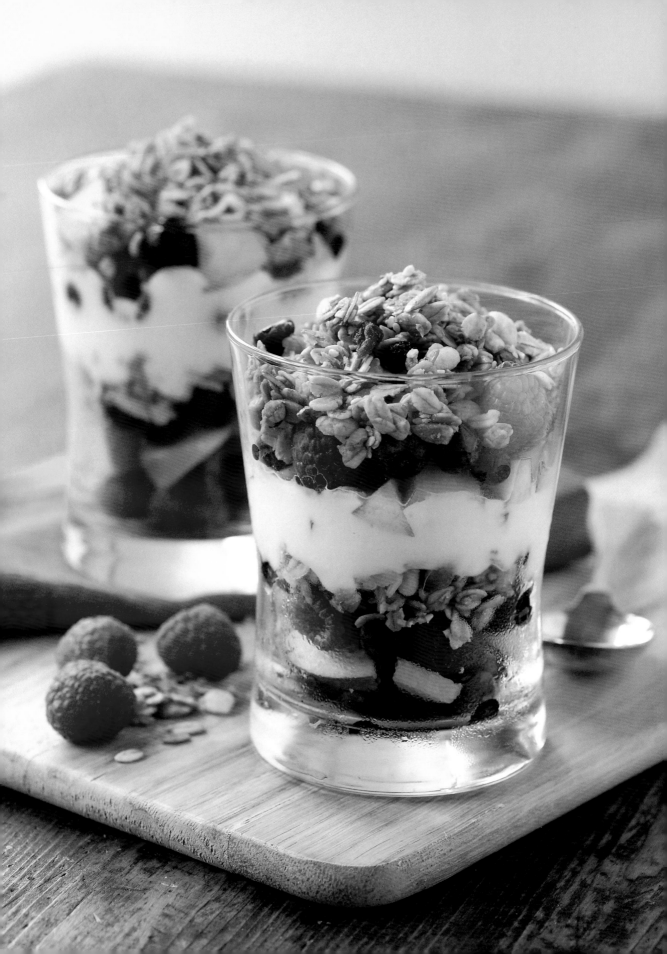

MAX'S BRANBERRY MUFFINS

Makes 1 dozen small muffins

PER SERVING
217 calories
5 g protein
6 g fat
37 g carbohydrate
5 g fiber
114 mg sodium

Chef's Secret

BUTTERMILK SUBSTITUTE If you don't have buttermilk on hand, make some by squeezing a few drops of lemon juice or white vinegar into regular milk and letting it sit for a few minutes.

Our grandson, Max, adores these muffins. I always have some on hand in the freezer for his visits as they freeze beautifully. Midday food cravings? Add a muffin to your lunch kit for a nutritious and delicious treat.

¾ cup (175 mL) brown sugar

¾ cup (175 mL) whole wheat flour

½ cup (125 mL) all-purpose flour

½ cup (125 mL) whole wheat bran

¼ cup (60 mL) wheat germ

1 tsp (5 mL) baking soda

1 cup (250 mL) blueberries, fresh or frozen

½ cup (125 mL) seedless raisins

1 Tbsp (15 mL) orange zest

⅔ cup (150 mL) plus 2 to 3 Tbsp (30 to 45 mL) reduced-fat buttermilk

1 large egg

¼ cup (60 mL) vegetable oil

Preheat the oven to 400°F (200°C) and lightly grease a small-sized 12-cup muffin pan with vegetable oil. Mix together the brown sugar, whole wheat flour, all-purpose flour, bran, wheat germ and baking soda in a large bowl. Stir in the blueberries, raisins and orange zest. Whisk ⅔ cup (150 mL) of the buttermilk with the egg and oil in a separate bowl. Add to the dry ingredients all at once, mixing well. Add 2 to 3 Tbsp (30 to 45 mL) more buttermilk if necessary to bind the batter. Spoon ¼ cup (60 mL) of batter into each muffin cup and bake about 20 minutes or until a skewer inserted in center of the muffin comes out clean. Serve immediately. Or set aside and reheat in aluminum foil in oven at 400°F (200°C) about 5 to 8 minutes. To freeze, put in plastic bags, seal and freeze for up to 3 months. Never microwave to reheat.

JEN'S POWER MUFFINS

Our daughter, Jennifer, perfected this muffin recipe when she was attending drama school in Toronto. They're an absolute fuel builder to start your day or for a midday snack. One muffin is all you need to satisfy your hunger.

4 large eggs, slightly beaten

4 cups (1 L) mashed ripe bananas (about 6 large bananas)

1⅓ cups (325 mL) vegetable oil

1 cup (250 mL) reduced-fat buttermilk

¾ cup (175 mL) brown sugar

1 Tbsp (15 mL) vanilla

1 cup (250 mL) chopped apricots

1 cup (250 mL) chopped dates

1 cup (250 mL) chopped prunes

1 cup (250 mL) dried cranberries

1 cup (250 mL) raisins

⅓ cup (75 mL) toasted sunflower seeds

⅓ cup (75 mL) flax seeds

2 cups (500 mL) all-purpose flour

2 cups (500 mL) whole wheat flour

1¼ cups (310 mL) wheat bran

¾ cup (175 mL) wheat germ

4 tsp (20 mL) baking powder

4 tsp (20 mL) baking soda

2 tsp (10 mL) cinnamon

¾ tsp (4 mL) nutmeg

sunflower seeds for garnish

Makes about 1½ dozen large or 2 dozen medium-sized muffins

PER SERVING
338 calories
7 g protein
15 g fat
47 g carbohydrates
7 g fiber
172 mg sodium

Chef's Secret
MUFFINS IN THE FREEZER These muffins freeze very well. Once you make your first batch, you'll always want to have an extra batch in the freezer! When eating at home, I like to reheat them in aluminum foil in the oven 400°F (200°C) about 5 to 8 minutes to serve warm. Never, but never, reheat them in a microwave; it can destroy their texture entirely.

Preheat the oven to 400°F (200°C) and lightly grease two 12-cup medium-sized muffin pans with vegetable oil. In a large bowl, combine the following and blend well: the eggs, mashed banana, vegetable oil, buttermilk, brown sugar and vanilla. Add the chopped apricots, dates, prunes, cranberries, raisins, sunflower seeds and flax seeds. In a separate bowl, blend the all-purpose flour, whole wheat flour, wheat bran, wheat germ, baking powder, baking soda, cinnamon and nutmeg. Fold the dry ingredients into the wet ingredients just to blend. Do not overbeat. Fill the prepared muffin cups to the top and sprinkle with a few additional sunflower seeds. Bake about 25 to 30 minutes, or until a skewer inserted in center of the muffin comes out clean. The muffin batter will keep in the refrigerator for up to 2 days, and the baked muffins will keep moist for the same amount of time.

DIANE'S ENERGY COOKIES

Makes 2½ to 3 dozen

PER SERVING
220 calories
7 g protein
14 g fat
18 g carbohydrate
4 g fiber
34 mg sodium

Chef's Secret

HAVE YOU HAD YOUR SEEDS TODAY? Sunflower seeds are rich in protein, iron and vitamins B and E. They also contain zinc, which is necessary for a healthy reproductive system, healthy skin and the immune system, and potassium, which regulates body fluids. Just ¼ cup (60 mL) of sunflower seeds contributes more than 90% of the recommended daily intake of vitamin E. For an added crunch, toast sunflower seeds on a baking sheet in a 350°F (180°C) oven about 5 or 6 minutes or until golden. Roasting the seeds will enhance their storage time.

These giant cookies are an excellent energy booster at breakfast, or any other time of day, so pack them in bag lunches, picnic baskets and hiking backpacks. Forget those expensive commercially prepared energy bars. These cookies get rave reviews.

1 cup (250 mL) whole wheat flour

2 tsp (10 mL) cinnamon

1 tsp (5 mL) baking powder

¼ tsp (1 mL) ground ginger

½ cup (125 mL) raisins

½ cup (125 mL) chopped dried cherries

½ cup (125 mL) chopped dried cranberries

1 cup (250 mL) regular oatmeal (not instant)

1 cup (250 mL) chopped toasted walnuts

1 cup (250 mL) chopped toasted pecans

1 cup (250 mL) unsalted peanuts

½ cup (125 mL) toasted sunflower seeds

½ cup (125 mL) toasted sesame seeds (page 97)

½ cup (125 mL) wheat germ

1¼ cup (310 mL) peanut butter

¼ cup (60 mL) unsalted butter

1 cup (250 mL) brown sugar

2 large eggs

¼ cup (60 mL) skim milk

Preheat the oven to 350°F (180°C) and lightly grease a baking sheet with vegetable oil. Combine the flour, cinnamon, baking powder and ginger in a large bowl. Add the raisins, cherries and cranberries and toss until coated. Add the oatmeal, nuts, seeds and wheat germ and mix together. In a separate bowl, cream together the peanut butter and butter. Add the sugar and beat well, and then add 1 egg at a time. Add the skim milk. Pour the butter mixture over the dry ingredients, and stir well or mix with your hands until the dry ingredients are well moistened. Drop by heaping tablespoons 3 inches (7 cm) apart on the prepared baking sheet. Flatten cookies slightly. Bake on the second rack from the bottom of the oven for 15 to 18 minutes, until light brown and semi-firm to touch. Transfer cookies to wire rack to cool. They keep fresh for several days.

MUSHROOM *and* CHEESE STRATA

Strata, bread pudding or bread soufflé—whatever you call it—dates back to the early settlers. This comfort food has recently come full circle by making a major comeback. Serve with Roasted Tomatoes (page 145).

1 cup (250 mL) grated Emmenthal or Gruyère cheese, or a combination of both

1½ cups (375 mL) grated Parmesan cheese

2 Tbsp (30 mL) olive oil

4 cups (1 L) white or crimini mushrooms, sliced

½ cup (125 mL) thin julienne strips of leek (white parts only), coarsely chopped

½ cup (125 mL) coarsely chopped shallots or white onions

1 Tbsp (15 mL) olive oil

6 large eggs

3 cups (750 mL) skim milk

2 tsp (10 mL) Dijon mustard

freshly ground pepper to taste

½ tsp (2 mL) Spanish sweet paprika

10 cups (2.5 L) whole wheat French bread, crustless and cubed

Serves 8

PER SERVING
429 calories
27 g protein
19 g fat
37 g carbohydrate
5 g fiber
912 mg sodium

Chef's Secret

Try substituting low-fat cheddar or Monterey Jack for the Gruyère cheese. Or try enhancing the flavor by adding ½ lb (250 g) of cubed baked ham or cooked cubed chicken. For brunch, serve with whole wheat bagels, low-fat cream cheese and a platter of fresh fruit. For dinner, serve the strata as a side dish instead of potatoes with meat or chicken.

THE DAY BEFORE Mix together the Emmenthal cheese with 1 cup (250 mL) of the grated Parmesan cheese. Set aside.

Warm 1 Tbsp (15 mL) of the olive oil in a frying pan over low to medium heat. Add the mushrooms and sauté for a few minutes, until softened. Set aside. Add the remaining 1 Tbsp (15 mL) of olive oil and sauté the leeks and shallots for a few minutes, until softened. Add to the mushrooms and set aside.

Combine the eggs, milk, mustard, pepper and paprika in a mixing bowl and whisk well to blend.

Lightly grease a 13- by 9-inch (3.5 L) casserole dish with vegetable oil. Layer one-third of the bread, followed by one-third of the cheese mixture and then one-third of the mushroom mixture. Repeat layers 2 times.

Pour the egg and milk mixture evenly over the casserole, and press down lightly. Cover and refrigerate for 6 to 8 hours or overnight.

DAY OF SERVING Remove from refrigerator about 1 hour before baking. Preheat the oven to 350°F (180°C). Sprinkle the remaining ½ cup (125 mL) grated Parmesan cheese evenly over the top. Bake 50 to 60 minutes, or until a knife comes out clean. It should be puffy and golden on top.

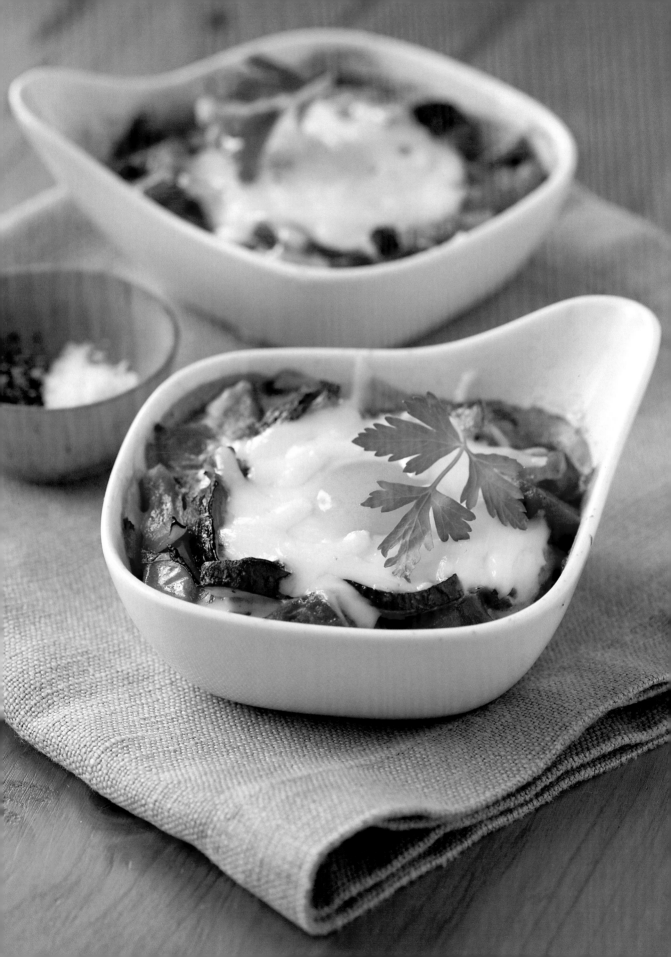

EGGS *with* QUICK RATATOUILLE

Ratatouille is a versatile side dish for chicken, meat and seafood. For an easy weekend brunch, it's a tasty base for eggs. Make the ratatouille 1 to 2 days ahead, then, on the morning of your brunch, top with eggs, bake and serve. It's as easy as that! Serve with warmed whole wheat tortillas. Ratatouille freezes well. Take out of the freezer the night before and refrigerate.

Serves 8

PER SERVING
200 calories
10 g protein
9 g fat
21 g carbohydrate
6 g fiber
150 mg sodium

QUICK RATATOUILLE

1 Tbsp (15 mL) vegetable oil

½ cup (125 mL) chopped onions

2 cloves of garlic, finely chopped

1 medium eggplant, cored, peeled and cubed ½ inch (1 cm)

¼ cup (60 mL) tomato juice or 2 Tbsp (30 mL) tomato paste

1 red pepper, seeded and diced

1 yellow pepper, seeded and diced

1 lb (500 g) zucchini, ends trimmed and then sliced ¼ inch (6 mm) thick

½ cup (125 mL) finely chopped fresh Italian parsley

3 Tbsp (45 mL) each of chopped fresh basil and fresh oregano

pinch of red pepper flakes

freshly ground pepper to taste

3 or 4 large tomatoes, peeled, seeded and cubed

EGGS

8 large eggs

½ cup (125 mL) grated low-fat Monterey Jack cheese

½ cup (125 mL) finely chopped Italian parsley

Chef's Secret

BRUNCH BASICS There's something totally relaxing about a long leisurely weekend brunch. Invite your friends over around 11 a.m. and expect them to leave around 3 p.m. No one will be in a rush. Keep it simple with Eggs with Quick Ratatouille or follow the Santa Fe Brunch menu (page 56).

FULL-OF-FLAVOR RATATOUILLE PASTA Add ratatouille to cooked pasta and sprinkle with a little Parmesan. It also goes great with grilled or steamed fish. Try snapper, sablefish, salmon or halibut.

1 OR 2 DAYS BEFORE Preheat the oven to 400°F (200°C). Warm the oil in a large frying pan over medium heat. Sauté the onions and garlic until softened. Add the eggplant and tomato juice. Cook about 5 minutes uncovered until softened, stirring from time to time. Add the peppers, zucchini and herbs. Cook a few minutes and then add the tomatoes. Simmer a few minutes more. Spoon into a 13- by 9-inch (3.5 L) casserole dish. Cover and bake 20 to 25 minutes. Cool, cover and refrigerate for 2 to 3 days, or freeze in containers.

DAY OF SERVING Take ratatouille casserole out of refrigerator and preheat the oven to 400°F (200°C). When oven is ready, warm the ratatouille about 20 to 30 minutes, or until very hot and bubbly. The heat is important for the baking of the eggs. Make 8 large indentations in the ratatouille mixture with the back of a large spoon, spacing them evenly. Break an egg into each indentation. Sprinkle the cheese over all. Bake 7 to 10 minutes, or until the whites are set but the yolks are still runny. Sprinkle with the parsley and serve.

SANTA FE CORN PIE

Serves 6

PER SERVING
225 calories
10 g protein
8 g fat
24 g carbohydrate
1 g fiber
470 mg sodium

Children love this pie. You could call it another do-ahead lifesaver as it works well for brunch or dinner. Add a tossed side salad and your meal is complete.

3 large eggs

1 cup (250 mL) canned cream-style corn

one 10 oz (284 mL) package frozen corn, thawed, or 1½ cups (375 mL) canned corn niblets, drained

½ cup (125 mL) 100% stone-ground wholegrain yellow cornmeal

1 cup (250 mL) fat-free sour cream

¼ cup (60 mL) grated low-fat Monterey Jack cheese

one 4 oz (113 g) can chopped mild green chilies

freshly ground pepper to taste

¼ tsp (1 mL) Worcestershire sauce

¼ tsp (1 mL) Tabasco sauce

3 Tbsp (45 mL) chopped green onions

Preheat the oven to 350°F (180°C) and lightly grease a 10-inch (25 cm) pie or quiche plate with vegetable oil. Whisk the eggs together in a large bowl. Add the creamed corn, corn niblets, cornmeal, sour cream, cheese, chilies, pepper, Worcestershire sauce, Tabasco and green onions and stir until thoroughly mixed. Pour into the prepared pie plate and bake uncovered about 45 to 50 minutes, or until golden and firm in the middle. The pie may be baked ahead and refrigerated for up to 3 days, or frozen.

TO REHEAT Preheat the oven to 350°F (180°C) and heat about 20 to 25 minutes, or until warmed. To reheat 1 piece, microwave about 1½ to 2 minutes, or until heated through.

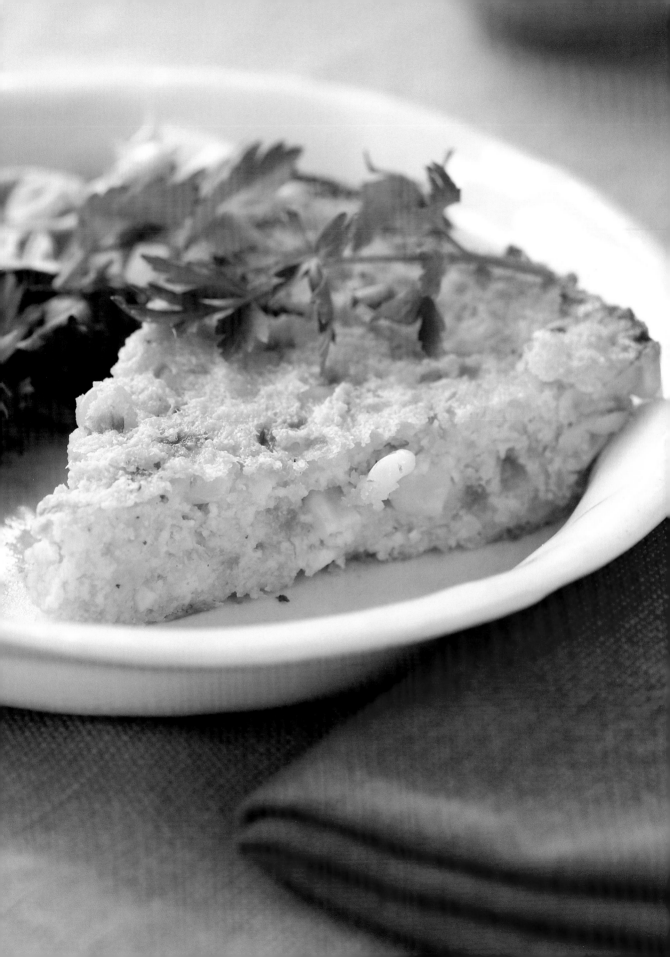

soup's on

MAUI SWEET ONION SOUP *with* SUN-DRIED TOMATO CHÈVRE CROSTINI

Our family has enjoyed many relaxed vacations at Bill and Gerry Gartside's Maui retreat. There we often dined at celebrity chef Yamaguchi's superb restaurants to enjoy his innovative Hawaiian cuisine. His sweet onion soup, a lighter version of the classic French onion soup, is so simple and refreshing. This is my take on his quick-to-make onion soup. It's a delightful starter course for Jane's Grilled Tuna Salad with Mango Pineapple Salad (page 93). Make this soup 1 to 2 days before serving so that the flavors have time to develop.

MAUI SWEET ONION SOUP

2 tsp (10 mL) olive oil

3 sweet onions, peeled, cut in half and sliced paper thin (about 2½ cups/625 mL)

2 large cloves of garlic, crushed

6 cups (1.5 L) low-sodium chicken stock

freshly ground pepper to taste

SUN-DRIED TOMATO CHÈVRE CROSTINI

12 Crostini (page 161)

½ cup (125 mL) chèvre (goat cheese)

6 sun-dried tomatoes in oil, finely chopped

2 Tbsp (30 mL) finely chopped fresh basil

¼ cup (60 mL) grated Parmesan cheese for garnish

Serves 6

PER SERVING
380 calories
16 g protein
11 g fat
48 g carbohydrate
1 g fiber
28 mg sodium

Chef's Secret
ONE SWEET ONION
Maui onions are next to impossible to find, but when in season, Walla Walla onions from Washington State or Vidalia onions from Georgia are superb for this soup recipe. Otherwise, any sweet onion will do. Use a mandolin to slice the onions easily.

1 OR 2 DAYS BEFORE Prepare the onion soup. Warm the oil in a medium-sized pot over medium heat. Add the onions and garlic. Turn the heat to low and sauté until golden and softened, about 10 to 15 minutes, stirring frequently. Add the stock; simmer uncovered 25 to 30 minutes. Add the pepper. Cool and then refrigerate.

THE DAY BEFORE Make the Crostini.

Prepare the Sun-Dried Tomato Chèvre. Blend together the chèvre, sun-dried tomatoes and basil in a small bowl, cover and refrigerate overnight.

JUST BEFORE SERVING Preheat the oven to 375°F (190°C). Warm the soup over medium heat. While the soup is heating, assemble the Sun-Dried Tomato Chèvre Crostini. Place the 12 crostini on a baking sheet and spread about 2 tsp (10 mL) of the chèvre mixture on each one. Sprinkle a little of the Parmesan cheese overtop. Place on the baking sheet and bake a few minutes to warm.

TO SERVE Ladle the soup into 6 small bowls. Top each bowl with 2 crostini.

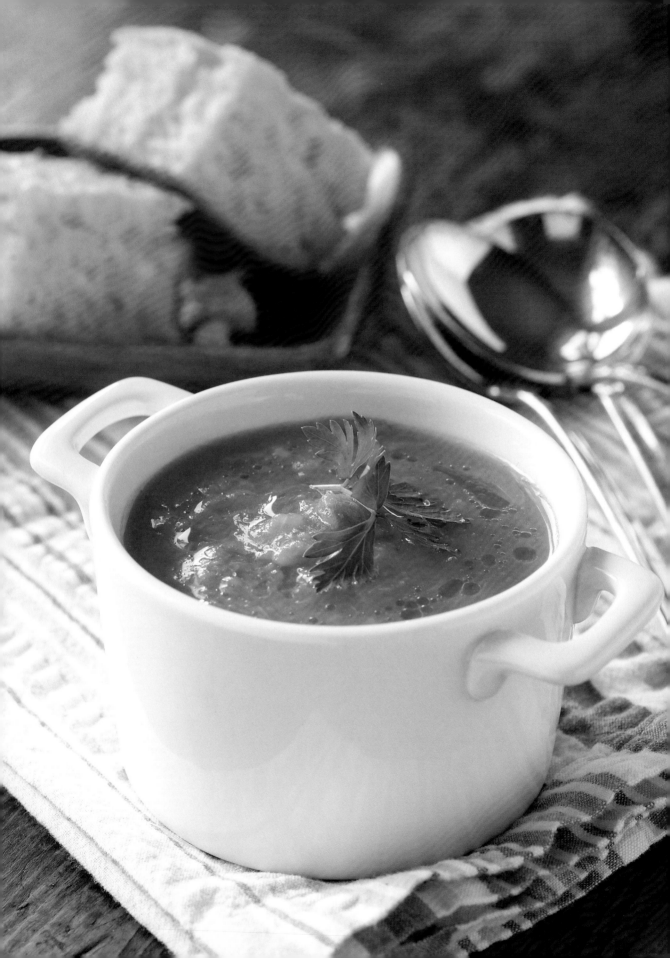

CARROT TOMATO SOUP

This is a favorite family recipe that I double-batch and freeze so I can pull it out any time of year. The difference with this version is that I have cut out the butter and substituted a little olive oil, and used low-fat and low-sodium chicken stock. And would you believe that a bowl of this soup boasts only 80 calories, chock full of garden-fresh flavors? Who needs a soup laden with butter and cream? If it seems too thick, thin it with chicken stock or tomato juice.

YOGURT PESTO TOPPING   *Makes ½ cup (125 mL)*

¼ cup (60 mL) low-fat yogurt

¼ cup (60 mL) basil pesto

CARROT TOMATO SOUP

4 tsp (20 mL) olive oil

3 medium-sized carrots, peeled and shredded

½ large onion, chopped

1 large leek, white part only, cleaned and chopped

1 clove of garlic, finely chopped

freshly ground pepper to taste

½ tsp (2 mL) ground coriander

½ tsp (2 mL) cumin

¼ tsp (1 mL) turmeric

pinch of red pepper flakes

2 large potatoes, peeled and coarsely chopped

4 cups (1 L) low-fat and low-sodium chicken stock

3 large tomatoes, peeled, seeded and chopped

one 14 oz (398 mL) can tomatoes, including juice

CONTINUED ON NEXT PAGE

Makes about 8 cups (2 L), enough to serve 6

PER SERVING

80 calories

3 g protein

2 g fat

14 g carbohydrate

2 g fiber

160 mg sodium

Chef's Secret

PEELING TOMATOES   To peel and seed tomatoes, slice an X on the bottom of the tomatoes and cut out the cores. Place the tomatoes in a bowl and pour boiling water over them to cover. Leave for 1 minute or until the skin starts to shrink. Cut in half horizontally and peel off the skin. Squeeze out the seeds and chop the flesh.

1 OR 2 DAYS BEFORE Blend the yogurt and pesto in a small bowl. Cover and refrigerate.

THE DAY BEFORE Warm the olive oil in a large pot over medium heat. Add the carrots, onion, leek, garlic, pepper, coriander, cumin and turmeric and red pepper flakes. Sauté for a few minutes until the onions are soft. Add the potatoes and 2 cups (500 mL) of the chicken stock. Bring to a boil, cover and cook over low heat, stirring frequently, about 10 minutes. Be careful the soup doesn't stick to the bottom of the pan.

Add the remaining stock and the tomatoes. Bring back to a boil and simmer, with lid askew, about 25 to 30 minutes, or until the potatoes are cooked. Cool. Purée in a food processor in small batches. The mixture should be slightly chunky.

Leave overnight in the refrigerator to allow the flavors to meld. To freeze, ladle the soup into 2-cup (500 mL) plastic containers and freeze for up to 3 months.

TO SERVE If frozen, thaw overnight in the refrigerator. Reheat until very hot, stirring frequently to blend ingredients. Ladle into soup bowls. Top with a small spoonful of the yogurt pesto topping and swirl with a knife.

GAZPACHO

One of the food delights that I look forward to when summer rolls around is making batches of Gazpacho, the traditional cold Spanish soup. It's healthy and refreshing, and with only 63 calories a cup, it's the perfect choice to ward off hunger cravings at any time of day. Try taking it to work for lunch or serve it as a starter course at dinner. I call it my liquid salad with zing. Make a large batch days in advance because this soup improves with age, although around our house, I must admit it disappears quickly.

Serves 12 to 16

PER SERVING
63 calories
2 g protein
1 g fat
12 g carbohydrate
2 g fiber
167 mg sodium

4 cups (1 L) chopped ripe tomatoes (about 8 large)

one 14 oz (398 mL) can tomatoes

½ onion, chopped

2 English cucumbers, peeled and chopped

2 red peppers, seeded and chopped

2 cups (500 mL) vegetable juice

2 cups (500 mL) tomato juice

4 sprigs of Italian parsley

2 cloves of garlic, finely chopped

½ cup (125 mL) Heinz-10 chili sauce

¼ cup (60 mL) chopped basil

¼ cup (60 mL) chopped dill

juice of 1 lemon

1 Tbsp (15 mL) white wine vinegar

½ tsp (2 mL) Spanish or Hungarian sweet paprika

½ tsp (2 mL) Worcestershire sauce

freshly ground pepper to taste

Croutons (page 160) for garnish

chopped green onions for garnish

AT LEAST 2 TO 3 DAYS BEFORE Cut the ripe tomatoes, canned tomatoes, onion, cucumbers and peppers into chunks. Put them through a food processor with the vegetable juice, tomato juice, parsley and garlic, processing a portion at a time, with on-off motions. Add the chili sauce, basil, dill, lemon juice, vinegar, paprika, Worcestershire sauce and pepper and blend slightly. Do not overprocess; keep the mixture chunky. If you prefer a thinner soup, add more tomato juice and experiment with the herbs and seasonings until the soup is to your liking. Cover and refrigerate for up to 4 to 5 days.

TO SERVE Ladle into small bowls and pass the Croutons and green onions.

from the garden

Salads and Salad Dressings

TOMATO, RED ONION
and WHITE BEAN SALAD

Great for a summertime barbecue or to include in an Italian antipasto presentation.

Serves 4 to 6

PER SERVING
183 calories
4 g protein
10 g fat
19 g carbohydrate
7 g fiber
231 mg sodium

DRESSING

¼ cup (60 mL) lemon juice

1 tsp (5 mL) Dijon mustard

freshly ground pepper to taste

¼ cup (60 mL) olive oil

SALAD

one 14 oz (398 g) can cannellini beans, drained

⅓ cup (75 mL) finely chopped red onion

¼ cup (60 mL) chopped Italian parsley

4 Roma tomatoes, finely diced, or 8 cherry tomatoes, sliced in half

1 yellow or orange pepper, seeded and cut into thin julienne strips

2 cloves of garlic, finely chopped

UP TO 1 WEEK AHEAD Prepare the dressing. Whisk together the lemon juice, mustard and pepper in a small bowl, adding the olive oil slowly. Cover and refrigerate for up to 1 week.

SEVERAL HOURS BEFORE SERVING Combine the beans, onion, parsley, tomatoes, pepper and garlic in a medium-sized bowl. Drizzle with the dressing and toss together. Cover and refrigerate until ready to serve.

Chef's Secret

NIÇOISE VARIATION Place the Tomato, Red Onion and White Bean Salad on a large platter and add one 6 oz (175 g) can of tuna or Grilled Tuna (page 93). Sprinkle with niçoise or kalamata olives over the platter, add a few hard-boiled eggs and you have a colorful twist on the classic French *salade niçoise*.

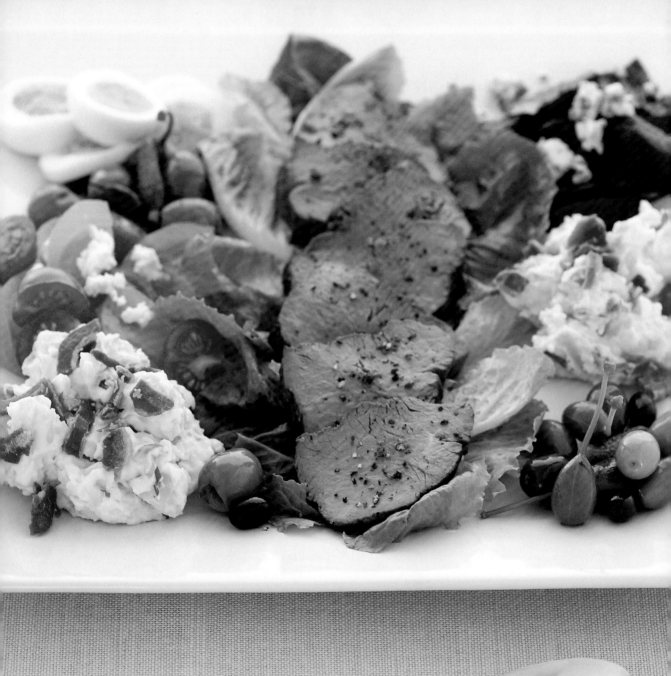
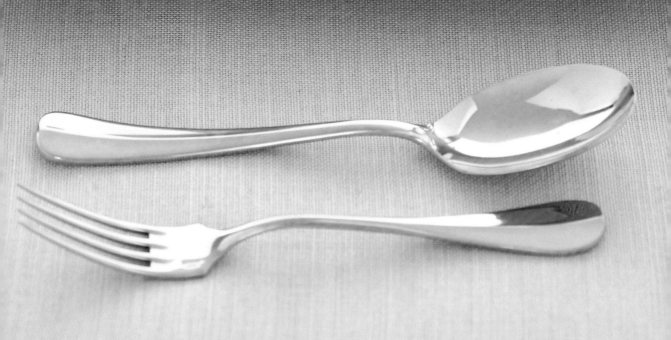

COBB SALAD ST. TROPEZ

This salad marries the popular American Cobb Salad with the French *salade niçoise*, an interesting match indeed. It's the perfect do-ahead for a family celebration (see Doug's July Birthday Celebration menu on page 55) so don't be intimidated by the salad prep. It takes a little time, but most of it can be done 1 to 2 days ahead, which is super for the host. Serve with warmed baguettes.

COBB SALAD DRESSING

2¼ cups (560 mL) Hellman's low-fat mayonnaise

¾ cup (175 mL) reduced-fat buttermilk

¾ cup (175 mL) grated Parmesan cheese

⅓ cup (75 mL) lemon juice

⅓ cup (75 mL) finely chopped green onions

1½ Tbsp (22 mL) Dijon mustard

dash of Worcestershire sauce

freshly ground pepper to taste

COBB SALAD

Grilled Lemon Chicken with Red Pepper or Fillet of Beef (recipe next page) Chutney (page 171)

4 cups (1 L) Potato Salad (recipe next page)

6 large hard-boiled eggs

6 oz (175 g) thinly sliced pancetta

3 cups (750 mL) Beet Salad (recipe next page)

3 cups (750 mL) cherry tomatoes, cut in half, or local heirloom tomatoes, sliced in quarters

4 cups (1 L) hearts of romaine or iceberg lettuce, torn in bite-sized pieces (about 2 heads)

1 cup (250 mL) niçoise or kalamata olives

1 cup (250 mL) Picholine olives or Italian green olives

¾ cup (175 mL) chèvre (goat cheese)

¾ cup (175 mL) crumbled blue cheese

CONTINUED ON NEXT PAGE

Serves 8

BASIC COBB SALAD

PER SERVING

330 calories

18 g protein

15 g fat

33 g carbohydrate

5 g fiber

750 mg sodium

COBB SALAD DRESSING

PER SERVING

142 calories

1 g protein

10 g fat

9 g carbohydrate

0 g fiber

483 mg sodium

PANCETTA

ADDS, PER SERVING

55 calories

7 g protein

3 g fat

0 g carbohydrate

0 g fiber

454 mg sodium

FILLET OF BEEF

ADDS, PER SERVING

290 calories

34 g protein

16 g fat

0 g carbohydrate

0 g fiber

80 mg sodium

GRILLED LEMON CHICKEN

ADDS, PER SERVING

195 calories

37 g protein

4 g fat

0 g carbohydrate

0 g fiber

87 mg sodium

POTATO SALAD

4 cups (1 L) baby red or white potatoes	
¾ cup (175 mL) Cobb Salad Dressing (recipe page 85)	
½ cup (125 mL) finely chopped green onions	
pinch of salt	
freshly ground pepper to taste	

FILLET OF BEEF

one 2 lb (1 kg) fillet of beef	
3 Tbsp (45 mL) grainy mustard	
freshly ground pepper to taste	
2 Tbsp (30 mL) olive oil	

BEET SALAD

3 cups (750 mL) Rand's Roasted Beets with Yogurt (page 130), sliced in small wedges	
1 Tbsp (15 mL) olive oil	
juice of ½ lemon	
3 Tbsp (45 mL) chopped Italian parsley	
freshly ground pepper to taste	

Chef's Secret

SHRIMP AND ICEBERG LETTUCE COBB SALAD Try the Cobb Salad Dressing on a wedge of crisp iceberg lettuce sprinkled with slices of avocados, cherry tomatoes sliced in half and fresh baby shrimp. Love it!

ABOUT PANCETTA
Pancetta is a cured but unsmoked Italian bacon. Since it's not smoked, it has a milder flavor than American bacon. The curing process is similar to that of prosciutto, where the hams are salted, then hung to air cure for at least 12 months.

1 OR 2 DAYS BEFORE Make the Cobb Salad Dressing. Combine the mayonnaise, buttermilk, lemon juice, Parmesan, mustard, Worcestershire sauce, green onions, and pepper in a small bowl. Cover and refrigerate.

Prepare the Grilled Lemon Chicken if you plan to serve it instead of the Fillet of Beef but omit the Red Pepper Chutney.

Prepare the Potato Salad. Boil the potatoes. Slice in halves, or quarters if larger. Add the dressing, onions, salt and pepper. Toss well. Cover and refrigerate.

Hard-boil the eggs. Cool and refrigerate.

SEVERAL HOURS BEFORE SERVING Prepare the Fillet of Beef (if using). Preheat the oven to 400°F (200°C). Rub the fillet all over with the mustard. Sprinkle with pepper. Warm the olive oil in a large frying pan over medium-high heat and sear the beef until evenly browned. Roast about 25 to 30 minutes, or until a meat thermometer reads 135°F (58°C) for medium rare. Do not overcook the beef! Remove from the oven and let sit until cooled. Cover and refrigerate.

Prepare the pancetta. Preheat the oven to 400°F (200°C). Lay the pancetta slices in an even layer on a baking sheet (you may have to use 2 baking sheets). Roast until crisp, about 12 to 15 minutes. Check after 8 minutes—turn the bacon over and pat dry with paper towels to remove the excess fat. When crisp, drain on paper towels. Set aside.

If using chicken, slice the Grilled Lemon Chicken into ¼-inch (6 mm) strips and refrigerate until you're ready to assemble the salad.

Peel the hard-boiled eggs and slice them in half. Cover and refrigerate.

Check the Potato Salad and add a little more dressing if the potatoes seem a bit dry, as they'll absorb the dressing overnight.

Prepare the Beet Salad. Combine all the ingredients in a bowl. Toss well. Cover and refrigerate.

Slice the tomatoes in half. Put in a bowl and leave at room temperature.

JUST BEFORE SERVING Tear the romaine into bite-sized pieces in a large salad bowl. Toss the romaine with enough dressing to coat well. Crumble the cooked pancetta over the salad and toss.

TO SERVE On a large salad platter, make a lettuce base in a row down the middle of the salad platter. Place the beef slices or chicken (if using) down the middle on top of the lettuce. Arrange everything else, except the cheeses, in colorful clusters on both sides of the beef. Now you can get creative in arranging the salad. Sprinkle the chèvre over the tomatoes and sprinkle the blue cheese over the beets. Place the platter in the middle of the table or buffet and let everyone help themselves. Pass the remaining dressing at the table, along with a couple of warmed baguettes.

ITALIAN MOZZARELLA *and* FENNEL SALAD

Serves 6

....

PER SERVING
325 calories
17 g protein
24 g fat
14 g carbohydrate
5 g fiber
430 mg sodium

Chef's Secret
BUFFALO MOZZARELLA
Mozzarella cheese was originally made only from buffalo milk, produced in the south of Italy. Buffalo mozzarella is more expensive and creamier than the factory-made version produced in the north of Italy from cow's milk. Buffalo mozzarella melts in your mouth and is the perfect marriage with tomatoes and fresh basil. Cow's milk mozzarella made in Italy or North America is popular on pizzas because of its melting quality.

This is a sensuous Tuscan salad that dates back to the 1800s. It was named Dama Bianca (Lady in White), because of its 3 white ingredients: fresh mozzarella, fennel and celery hearts. I've added orange segments to complement the licorice flavor of fennel. It's a sublime start to any Italian dinner that's well worth splurging on buffalo mozzarella from your cheese market. Serve with breadsticks and an Italian Pinot Grigio.

CITRUS VINAIGRETTE

¼ cup (60 mL) lemon juice

3 Tbsp (45 mL) orange juice

½ cup (125 mL) olive oil

freshly ground pepper to taste

SALAD

1 lb (500 g) buffalo mozzarella cheese balls or bocconcini

2 medium-sized fennel bulbs with fronds

3 celery hearts, white inner stalks only

¾ cup (175 mL) orange segments

THE DAY BEFORE Prepare the dressing. Blend the lemon and orange juices in a small bowl. Whisk in the olive oil and pepper. Cover and refrigerate.

DAY OF SERVING Thinly slice the mozzarella ball. Arrange in a circle in the middle of a salad platter.

Cut the fronds from the fennel and chop 3 Tbsp (45 mL) of fronds for the garnish. Set aside. Remove the tough outer sections of the fennel bulbs, cut the bulbs in half and remove the cores. Cut the remaining fennel into very thin julienne strips. Soak in a bowl of ice water about 10 minutes. Remove and pat dry.

Cut the leafy tops off the hearts of celery. Discard. Thinly slice the celery hearts on the diagonal. Soak in a bowl of ice water for 10 minutes. Remove and pat dry.

Scatter a layer of the fennel on top of the mozzarella and top with a layer of the celery hearts, finishing with a layer of the orange segments. Cover and refrigerate 1 or 2 hours before serving.

TO SERVE Drizzle enough citrus vinaigrette to glaze well. Sprinkle the salad with the chopped fennel fronds. Serve immediately. You can serve individual salad plates following the same method, using 1 thin mozzarella slice per plate.

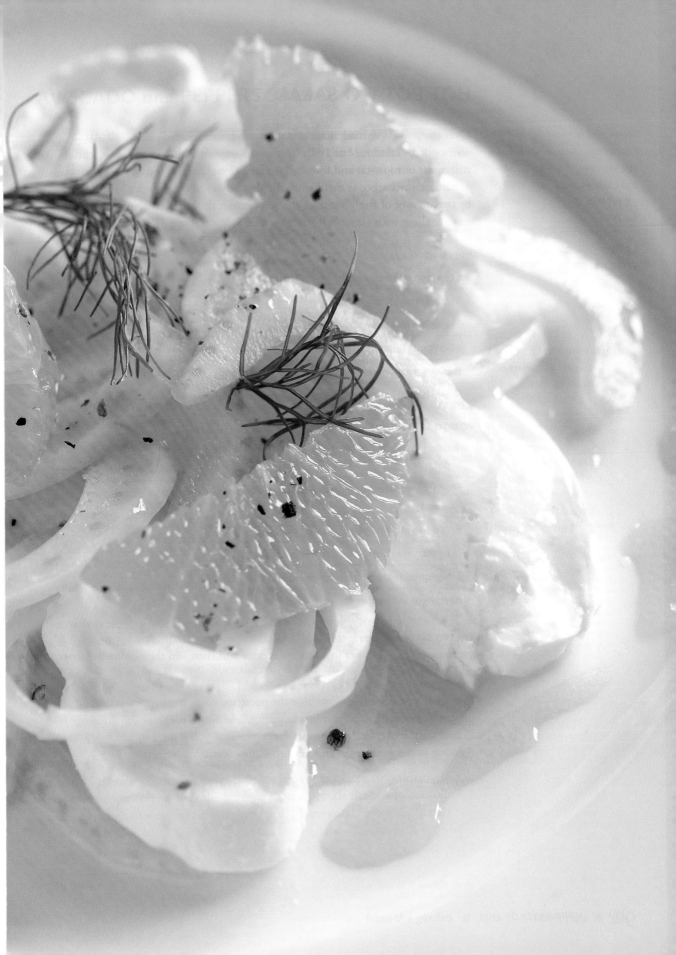

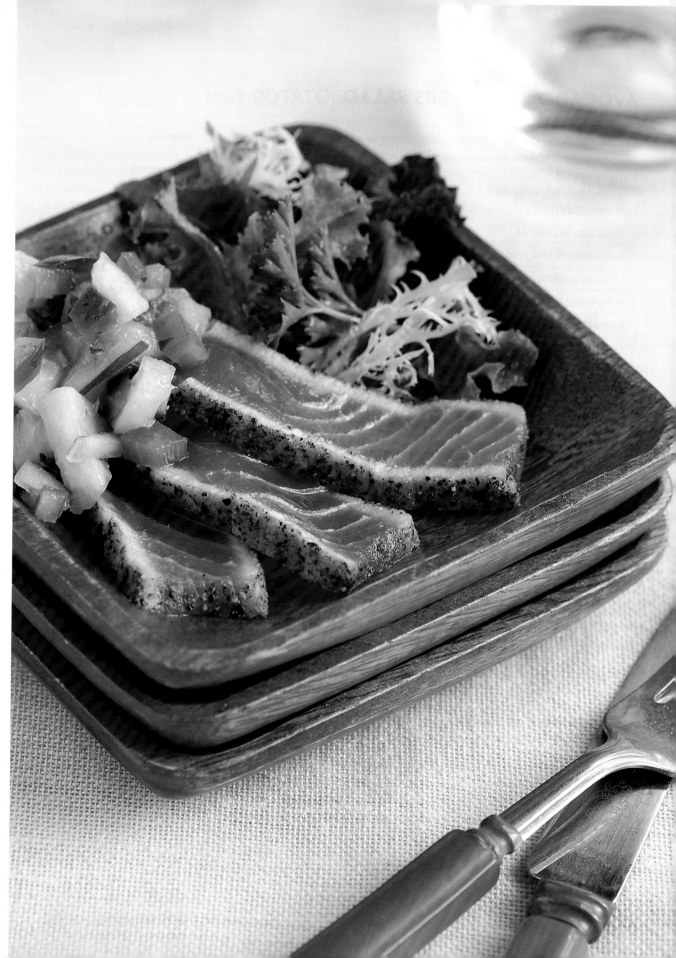

JANE'S GRILLED TUNA SALAD
with MANGO PINEAPPLE SALSA

During our stays in the Grand Cayman Islands at our friend Arden Shaw's beachfront home, we dined watching the spectacular sunsets. Jane MacDonald joined us on our holiday and raved over my tuna salad. This one's for you, Jane. I've included 2 different rubs for you to choose from to spice up the tuna: Pepper and Ginger Rub or Pepper, Sumac and Cumin Rub. The Maui Sweet Onion Soup (page 77) is the ideal starter course.

PEPPER AND GINGER RUB

2 Tbsp (30 mL) freshly ground pepper

2 Tbsp (30 mL) peeled and very finely chopped fresh ginger

PEPPER, SUMAC AND CUMIN RUB

¼ cup (60 mL) freshly ground pepper

1 Tbsp (15 mL) plus 1 tsp (5 mL) ground sumac, or 3 Tbsp (45 mL) lemon zest

½ tsp (2 mL) ground cumin

SALAD

4 cups (1 L) mixed greens

Ginger Lime Vinaigrette (page 104)

toasted white and black sesame seeds for garnish (page 97)

Mango Pineapple Salsa (page 111)

4 lime wedges for garnish

8 oz (200 g) sashimi-grade tuna

Pepper and Ginger Rub, or Pepper, Sumac and Cumin Rub

2 Tbsp (30 mL) olive or grape seed oil

CONTINUED ON NEXT PAGE

Serves 4

PER SERVING

240 calories

10 g protein

19 g fat

13 g carbohydrate

1 g fiber

640 mg sodium

Chef's Secret

TANGY SUMAC Sumac is a tart, lemony-flavored spice from the sumac berry bush and is used frequently in Eastern Mediterranean cuisines. I also like the Pepper, Sumac and Cumin Rub sprinkled on the Pita Crisps (page 159).

SEVERAL HOURS BEFORE SERVING Prepare the Pepper and Ginger Rub. In a small bowl, combine the ground pepper and ginger. Cover and refrigerate until ready to coat the tuna.

Alternatively, prepare the Pepper, Sumac and Cumin Rub. Combine the ground pepper, sumac and cumin in a small bowl. Place in a sealed jar and store in a cool place for up to 6 months. Substitute lemon zest for the sumac if it's unavailable.

JUST BEFORE SERVING Coat the tuna all over with either the Pepper and Ginger Rub or the Pepper, Sumac and Cumin Rub. Warm a little of the olive oil in a grill pan or barbecue over high heat. Grill the tuna about 2 minutes per side, just enough to sear the tuna on the outside and keep it rare on the inside. Set the tuna aside as you toss the greens.

Toss the mixed greens in a salad bowl with just enough Ginger Lime Vinaigrette to coat. Mound an equal amount on 4 salad plates. Slice the grilled tuna thinly and divide evenly, fan-shaped, on top of the greens. Drizzle a little dressing over the tuna slices. Sprinkle a few sesame seeds. Arrange a little of the Mango Pineapple Salsa on 1 side of the greens. Add a lime wedge on the other side. Pass more dressing and salsa at the table if desired.

ARUGULA *and* BLACK OLIVE SALAD

I love to serve this tart, refreshing salad with Mexican and Mediterranean dishes. Add a bit of protein with 2 cooked, cubed chicken breasts if desired.

VINAIGRETTE

⅓ cup (75 mL) lemon juice

2 Tbsp (30 mL) lemon zest

2 Tbsp (30 mL) chopped fresh mint

2 Tbsp (30 mL) chopped fresh oregano

2 tsp (10 mL) Dijon mustard

freshly ground pepper to taste

½ cup (125 mL) olive oil

SALAD

two 6 oz (175 g) bags of prewashed and dried arugula greens

2 ripe avocados, peeled and sliced

1½ cups (325 mL) kalamata olives, pitted and halved

½ cup (125 mL) crumbled chèvre (goat cheese) or feta cheese

THE DAY BEFORE Make the vinaigrette. Whisk together the lemon juice and zest, mint, oregano, mustard and pepper in a small bowl and slowly add the olive oil. Cover and refrigerate.

TO SERVE Put the greens in a large salad bowl. Add enough dressing just to coat. Toss lightly. Arrange on a large salad platter. Arrange the avocado slices on top of the arugula greens. Sprinkle the olives and cheese evenly over all. Drizzle with a little more vinaigrette. Serve immediately. Save any leftover dressing for another salad, as it stays fresh 2 to 3 days.

Serves 4 to 6

PER SERVING
300 calories
6 g protein
31 g fat
9 g carbohydrate
4 g fiber
280 mg sodium

Chef's Secret

STAY FRESH TIP Wrap fresh herbs in damp paper towels and store in a sealed plastic bag in the refrigerator. They will keep for 2 to 3 days. Chop herbs with a sharp knife or snip with scissors to prevent bruising the leaves.

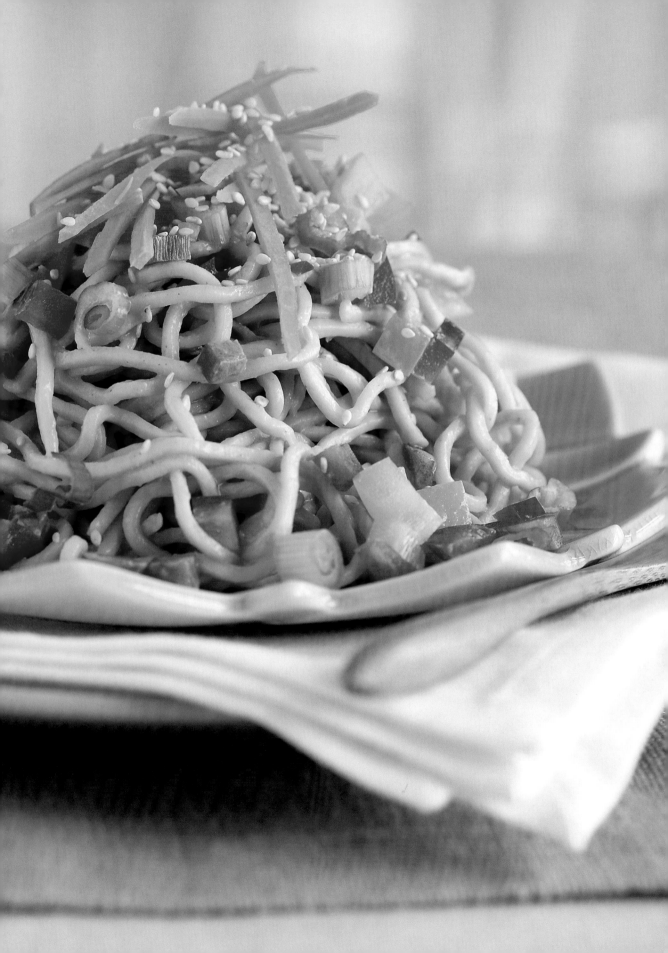

ASIAN NOODLE SALAD

This recipe is one of my classics. I've revised the original recipe to bring it in line with our healthy choices by substituting low-fat peanut butter for creamy peanut butter and low-sodium soy sauce for typically high-in-salt regular soy. This colorful salad is a small meal in itself and is best when made a day ahead. Buy the red pepper oil in the Asian food section of your supermarket or make your own.

DRESSING

½ cup (125 mL) low-fat peanut butter

¼ cup (60 mL) tamari

¼ cup (60 mL) low-sodium soy sauce

¼ cup (60 mL) rice wine vinegar or sherry vinegar

¼ cup (60 mL) red pepper oil

3 cloves of garlic

2 Tbsp (30 mL) sesame oil

RED PEPPER OIL

¼ cup (60 mL) vegetable oil

½ tsp (2 mL) red pepper flakes

SALAD

two 14 oz (398 g) packages steam-fried or dry chow mein noodles

2 Tbsp (30 mL) sesame oil

1 cup (250 mL) finely chopped and lightly blanched carrots

¾ cup (175 mL) finely chopped water chestnuts

½ cup (125 mL) finely chopped green onions

½ cup (125 mL) finely chopped red peppers

½ cup (125 mL) finely chopped yellow or orange peppers

½ cup (125 mL) finely chopped unsalted cashew nuts

3 Tbsp (45 mL) toasted sesame seeds (see sidebar)

CONTINUED ON NEXT PAGE

Serves 8

PER SERVING

680 calories

20 g protein

39 g fat

66 g carbohydrate

7 g fiber

700 mg sodium

Chef's Secret

SENSATIONAL SESAME SEEDS Toasted black and white sesame seeds can be found at specialty Asian shops. To toast your own sesame seeds, preheat the oven to 350°F (180°C). Spread the sesame seeds on a baking sheet and roast them about 5 minutes. Watch carefully or they'll burn and taste bitter.

UP TO 2 OR 3 DAYS BEFORE Prepare the dressing. Blend the peanut butter, tamari, soy sauce, vinegar, red pepper oil, garlic and sesame oil in a food processor until smooth. Cover and refrigerate. Any leftover dressing can be used as a sauce or dip for fish and meats.

To prepare your own red pepper oil, in a small saucepan combine the vegetable oil and red pepper flakes. Bring to a boil over medium heat and then remove immediately from the heat. Let sit for about 10 minutes. Strain into a sealed jar and store for up to 2 or 3 days. If you want a more intense flavor, let the peppers sit in the oil for 15 to 20 minutes longer before decanting.

THE DAY BEFORE Prepare the salad. Boil the noodles according to their directions; drain. Rinse well and toss with the sesame oil. Add the carrots, water chestnuts, green onions, red peppers, yellow peppers and cashew nuts and mix well. Add enough dressing to coat all the ingredients well. Cover and refrigerate overnight.

JUST BEFORE SERVING Add a little more dressing if the noodle salad seems too dry.

DIANE'S WESTCOASTER SALAD
with MAPLE BALSAMIC VINAIGRETTE

This Westcoaster Salad is totally a winner. When my daughter, Jennifer, and I opened the Tomato Fresh Food Café in 1991, this was our "Number One" salad. Now, new owners Christian Gaudreault and his wife, Starllie, still feature it on their menu, and it's as popular as ever. Whenever out-of-town guests come for dinner or lunch, I serve this salad. They all want the recipe to take home.

MAPLE BALSAMIC VINAIGRETTE

1 cup (250 mL) olive oil

¼ to ⅓ cup (60 to 75 mL) balsamic vinegar

¼ cup (60 mL) pure maple syrup

1 tsp (5 mL) Dijon mustard

freshly ground pepper to taste

SALAD

½ lb (250 g) peppered, candied, smoked salmon strips, or regular smoked salmon

6 cups (1.5 L) mixed greens

½ red pepper, seeded and cut into thin julienne strips

½ yellow pepper, seeded and cut into thin julienne strips

1 cup (250 mL) crumbled chèvre (goat cheese)

2 OR 3 DAYS BEFORE Prepare the Maple Balsamic Vinaigrette. Whisk together the olive oil, balsamic vinegar, maple syrup, mustard and pepper. Cover and refrigerate.

JUST BEFORE SERVING Peel the skin off the salmon, and slice diagonally into ¼-inch (6 mm) thick slices. Set aside.

Divide the greens evenly among 6 salad plates, mounding them high.

Warm the vinaigrette in a frying pan over low heat. Add the slices of salmon and the peppers. Heat briefly a few minutes to warm.

TO SERVE On each salad plate, divide the salmon mixture equally over the greens, then drizzle with the warm dressing. Top with a good sprinkling of chèvre. Serve immediately.

Serves 6

PER SERVING
335 calories
19 g protein
27 g fat
5 g carbohydrate
1 g fiber
217 mg sodium

Chef's Secret
PEPPERED, CANDIED SMOKED SALMON Look for this delicious version of smoked salmon in the seafood section of your local food and seafood markets. Candied smoked salmon is usually marinated with a little honey, maple syrup or dark brown sugar and a little salt. Coarsely ground pepper is sometimes added as well. It's smoked from 8 to 24 hours to give the salmon a sweet, subtle smoky flavor. It's slightly crusty on the outside, but moist and soft on the inside, not like the "Indian candy salmon" variety which is chewy. Choose nice thick strips. I always keep some on hand in the freezer. Take it out in the morning and thaw it in the refrigerator.

WATERMELON *and* OLIVE TAPENADE CARPACCIO SALAD

Chef's Secret

MAKE YOUR OWN DRESSING It's so easy to whip up an endless variety of dressings. I usually have at least 2 different choices in my refrigerator. Once you start making your own you won't enjoy the artificial taste of most commercially prepared dressings. Invest in good quality olive oil and vinegars. Save less expensive oils for cooking.

Remember that dressings add calories. Use just enough dressing to coat the salads; don't drown them.

I love to serve my guests this refreshing palate pleaser, either before or after the main course, or as an opening salad. Bring a basket of Italian breadsticks to the table.

LEMON VINAIGRETTE

juice of 1½ lemons

¼ cup (60 mL) olive oil

freshly ground pepper to taste

SALAD

1½ cups (375 mL) arugula greens, washed and dried

1 small round seedless watermelon

juice of 1 lime

freshly ground pepper to taste

½ cup (125 mL) black olive tapenade

½ cup (125 mL) chèvre (goat cheese) or feta cheese

6 large basil leaves

1 OR 2 DAYS BEFORE Prepare the Lemon Vinaigrette. Whisk together the lemon juice, olive oil and pepper in a small bowl. Cover and refrigerate.

TO SERVE Toss the arugula greens in a bowl with enough vinaigrette to coat. Divide the arugula evenly among 6 salad plates, placing the greens in the middle of each plate. Slice the watermelon in half. Cut each half into 4 wedges and remove the skin. Slice the wedges into ½-inch (1 cm) thick triangle slices, allowing 4 slices per person. Pat dry and arrange them on an angle on one side of the greens. Drizzle with the lime juice and a dash of pepper. Place 1 Tbsp (15 mL) of the olive tapenade on the opposite side of the watermelon. Sprinkle the chèvre evenly over all and place a basil leaf next to the tapenade. Serve immediately.

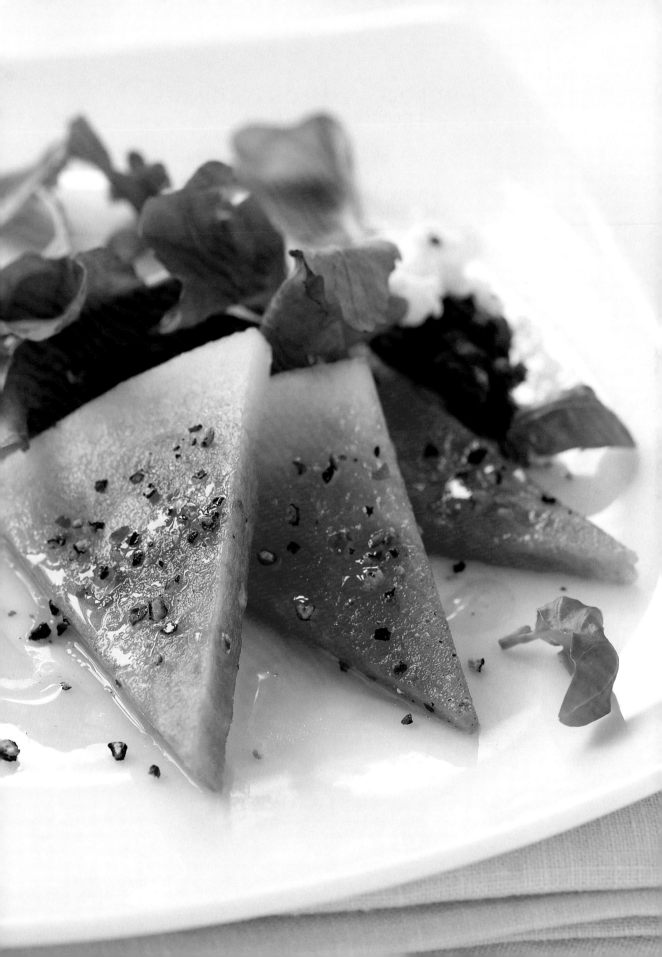

MOROCCAN MELON *and* GINGER FRUIT SALAD

Serves 6 to 8

....

PER SERVING
56 calories
1 g protein
0 g fat
15 g carbohydrate
1 g fiber
21 mg sodium

In Morocco, this refreshing fruit salad is usually served after the first course, before the tagine (stew). I like to serve a small portion in a martini glass. The secret is to put the salad in the freezer 10 minutes before serving so it's very chilled. I use my melon baller to prepare the fruit and allow about 5 melon balls per person. Any leftovers are delicious with low-fat yogurt. Make the day before so that the flavors blend.

LEMON GLAZE

juice of 2 lemons

2 Tbsp (30 mL) finely grated fresh ginger

1 Tbsp (15 mL) honey

SALAD

2 cups (500 mL) honeydew melon balls

2 cups (500 mL) cantaloupe balls

mint leaves for garnish

THE DAY BEFORE Prepare the Lemon Glaze by combining the lemon juice, ginger and honey in a medium bowl and set aside.

Make the melon balls and add them to the Lemon Glaze. Cover and refrigerate overnight.

TO SERVE Spoon the melon balls into martini glasses. Drizzle a little of the Lemon Glaze overtop and garnish with fresh mint leaves.

BASIC BALSAMIC VINAIGRETTE

¼ to ⅓ cup (60 to 75 mL) balsamic vinegar, or to taste

1 tsp (5 mL) Dijon mustard

freshly ground pepper to taste

1 cup (250 mL) olive oil

2 DAYS AHEAD Whisk together the vinegar, mustard and pepper until well blended, adding the olive oil slowly as the last ingredient. Add more vinegar and mustard if desired. Make at least 2 days ahead of serving for the flavors to develop. Dressing will keep in the refrigerator for up to 2 weeks.

Makes about 1¼ cups (310 mL)

PER 2 TSP (10 ML) SERVING
125 calories
0 g protein
14 g fat
1 g carbohydrate
0 g fiber
3 mg sodium

Chef's Secret
JAZZ UP THE BASIC BALSAMIC VINAIGRETTE
Add fresh herbs such as basil, oregano or dill, chopped green onions or shallots, Parmesan cheese or a little pesto to give more flavor to your dressings. Vary the vinaigrette by substituting a sherry, citrus, white or red wine vinegar for the balsamic vinegar. Or try the Maple Balsamic Vinaigrette (page 99).

GINGER LIME VINAIGRETTE

Makes about 1 cup (250 mL)

PER 2 TSP (10 ML) SERVING
130 calories
0 g protein
14 g fat
1 g carbohydrate
0 g fiber
154 mg sodium

Chef's Secret

NUTRITIOUS ADDITIONS
Add dried cranberries, fresh slices of mango, toasted almonds or pecans and/or thinly sliced peppers to the tossed greens when using this dressing.

This Asian flavored dressing is perfect for Jane's Grilled Tuna Salad with Mango Pineapple Salsa (page 93). Or try it on a simple tossed green salad.

3 Tbsp (45 mL) lime juice

2 Tbsp (30 mL) finely grated fresh ginger

2 Tbsp (30 mL) finely chopped shallots or green onions

2 Tbsp (30 mL) low-sodium soy sauce

2 Tbsp (30 mL) Chinese sweet chili sauce

1 Tbsp (15 mL) rice wine vinegar

1 clove of garlic, finely chopped

½ cup (125 mL) vegetable oil

1 Tbsp (15 mL) sesame oil

Whisk together the lime juice, ginger, shallots, soy sauce, chili sauce, vinegar and garlic in a small bowl. Slowly whisk in the vegetable oil and sesame oil. Cover and refrigerate for up to 1 week.

LOW-FAT CAESAR DRESSING

Now you can enjoy Caesar salad without feeling guilty. Add some whole wheat Croutons (page 160) and you have a winner. Add sliced chicken breasts or fresh baby shrimp to make this salad a meal in itself.

one 2 oz (50 g) can flat anchovy fillets in oil
1 Tbsp (15 mL) skim milk
½ cup (125 mL) Hellman's low-fat mayonnaise
4 tsp (20 mL) lemon juice
1½ tsp (7 mL) Worcestershire sauce
1½ tsp (7 mL) Dijon mustard
freshly ground pepper to taste

Drain the oil from the anchovies, wash and pat dry. Soak in the milk for a few minutes to take away the strong anchovy taste. Pat dry. Place the anchovies, mayonnaise, lemon juice, Worcestershire sauce, mustard and pepper in a food processor. Blend until very smooth, about 2 or 3 minutes. Cover and refrigerate for up to 2 to 3 days. Make at least 1 day ahead for the flavor to peak.

Makes ½ cup (125 mL)

PER 4 TSP (20 ML) SERVING
48 calories
1 g protein
3 g fat
5 g carbohydrate
0 g fiber
370 mg sodium

Chef's Secret
ANCHOVIES IN HIDING
You can usually find canned anchovies in the refrigerated dairy section of the grocery store. Keep refrigerated at home and use within 1 day of opening.

spice it up

Sauces, Salsas and Spice Mixes

ROASTED RED PEPPER SAUCE

This sauce is a perfect complement to the Pork Tenderloin Superb (page 167) or Fillet of Beef (page 86). Buy your roasted peppers at the deli or prepare them at home.

3 large roasted red peppers (see sidebar), washed and patted dry

⅓ cup (75 mL) finely chopped shallots

⅓ cup (75 mL) sherry vinegar

¼ cup (60 mL) soft chèvre (goat cheese)

2 garlic cloves, finely chopped

2 tsp (10 mL) balsamic vinegar

1 tsp (5 mL) Spanish sweet paprika

freshly ground pepper to taste

1 cup (250 mL) olive oil

1 OR 2 DAYS BEFORE Combine the red peppers, shallots, sherry vinegar, chèvre, garlic, balsamic vinegar, paprika and pepper in a food processor. Slowly add the olive oil to blend well and thicken. Cover and refrigerate.

TO SERVE Warm in a small saucepan over low heat, stirring constantly to keep smooth. Serve in a sauceboat with meats.

Makes about 2 cups (500 mL)

PER SERVING
280 calories
2 g protein
30 g fat
6 g carbohydrate
1 g fiber
23 mg sodium

Chef's Secret
ROASTING RED PEPPERS
Rub the peppers with a little olive oil. Roast them over a barbecue, hold them over a gas burner or broil them in the oven, turning them frequently until they're black and blistered all over. Put in a plastic bag and let cool. Remove from the bag and peel off the skin, which should come off easily. Remove the stalk, seeds and pith.

When you need only a few roasted peppers, pick them up from your deli. If you're using the pickled roasted peppers in jars, rinse them well as they tend to be very salty and sharp tasting. Any leftovers can be frozen and thawed as needed.

QUICK LEMON DILL MAYONNAISE

Makes about 1⅓ cups (325 mL)

....

PER SERVING
120 calories
1 g protein
5 g fat
24 g carbohydrate
1 g fiber
330 mg sodium

When time is short, reach for your low-fat mayonnaise and add seasonings. This mayonnaise goes well as a dip or spread with smoked salmon, grilled seafood or potato salad.

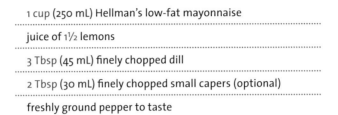

1 cup (250 mL) Hellman's low-fat mayonnaise
juice of 1½ lemons
3 Tbsp (45 mL) finely chopped dill
2 Tbsp (30 mL) finely chopped small capers (optional)
freshly ground pepper to taste

Combine the mayonnaise, lemon juice, dill, capers (if using) and pepper in a small bowl. Cover and refrigerate for up to 2 to 3 days.

ROASTED GARLIC AIOLI

Another shortcut to bring the flavors of France to your table is this modification of the Quick Lemon Dill Mayonnaise (see facing page). Serve with bouillabaisse, or with fresh prawns and crab.

juice of 1½ lemons

¼ tsp (1 mL) saffron threads

4 cloves of garlic

olive oil for coating

1 cup (250 mL) Hellman's low-fat mayonnaise

pinch cayenne

freshly ground pepper to taste

1 OR 2 DAYS BEFORE Mix the lemon juice and saffron threads and allow to sit while you roast the garlic. Preheat the oven to 350°F (180°C). Peel the garlic and toss it with a little olive oil just to coat. Wrap in aluminum foil and roast in the oven about 30 minutes or until softened. If the cloves are small, they'll roast more quickly, so check after 20 minutes. Cool and mash with a fork. Combine the mashed roasted garlic with the lemon and saffron mixture in a small bowl. Add the mayonnaise, cayenne and pepper. Cover and refrigerate for up to 2 to 3 days.

Makes about 1 cup (250 mL)

PER SERVING

130 calories

1 g protein

5 g fat

24 g carbohydrate

1 g fiber

330 mg sodium

Chef's Secret

MORE ROASTED GARLIC

If you enjoy roasted garlic, make lots. Slice the top off a whole head of garlic and rub with 1 tsp (5 mL) olive oil. Wrap in aluminum foil and roast at 350°F (180°C) about 30 to 35 minutes, or until soft (check with thin knife). Cool and then squeeze out the garlic onto crostini, pizza bases and risottos.

TOMATO *and* RED ONION SALSA

Makes 2½ cups (625 mL)

PER SERVING
10 calories
0 g protein
0 g fat
2 g carbohydrate
0 g fiber
2 mg sodium

Serve with the Tex-Mex Salmon Tacos (page 177) and other Mexican dishes.

2 cups (500 mL) peeled, seeded and chopped tomatoes

⅓ cup (75 mL) chopped red onions

2 Tbsp (30 mL) finely chopped cilantro

2 Tbsp (30 mL) finely chopped and seeded jalapeño chilies

1 Tbsp (15 mL) finely chopped fresh oregano

freshly ground pepper to taste

1 OR 2 HOURS BEFORE Combine the tomatoes, onions, cilantro, jalapeño, oregano and pepper in a medium-sized bowl. Cover with plastic wrap and store at room temperature until ready to use.

MANGO PINEAPPLE SALSA

In 1959, Doug and I drove from Vancouver to Acapulco on our honeymoon. The Pacific Highway was a rugged road in those days but we were young and adventurous. When we reached Acapulco, we stayed at Motel Ito, where they pampered us with authentic Mexican dinners under candlelight. Their salsas were fantastic. This one is perfect with grilled fish and chicken, freshly made and without the added preservatives of the commercial variety.

1 cup (250 mL) peeled, cored and diced pineapple
1 cup (250 mL) peeled, seeded and diced mangoes or papaya
½ cup (125 mL) finely chopped red onion
⅓ cup (75 mL) seeded and finely chopped red pepper
¼ cup (60 mL) seeded and finely chopped jalapeño or poblano pepper
¼ cup (60 mL) finely chopped mint or cilantro
2 Tbsp (30 mL) olive oil
2 Tbsp (30 mL) lime juice
1 Tbsp (15 mL) lime zest

Combine the pineapple, mangoes, onion, red pepper, jalapeño, mint, olive oil, lime juice and zest in a medium-sized bowl. Cover and refrigerate for up to 2 to 3 days.

Makes about 2½ cups (625 mL), enough to serve 6

PER SERVING
124 calories
2 g protein
0 g fat
32 g carbohydrate
4 g fiber
8 mg sodium

Chef's Secret

MEXICAN MANGOES The best mangoes to buy are the saffron-colored Ataufo variety from Mexico. They are smaller and juicier than their greener cousins. The flesh should yield to a light squeeze when they're ripe.

RAS-EL-HANOUT (MOROCCAN SPICE MIX)

PER SERVING
5 calories
0 g protein
0 g fat
1 g carbohydrate
0 g fiber
1 mg sodium

Chef's Secret

THE SULTAN'S SPICES: RAS-EL-HANOUT The Arabic name of this spice mix literally means "top of the grocer's shop." Every household and market has its own version of the spice blend, which can include 25 or more spices. No one will reveal their family secret for the spice blends passed down for generations. Some Middle Eastern delis carry ras-el-hanout, but if unavailable, mix up your own.

This Moroccan spice mix brings a delicate taste and fragrance to meat stews. It's used in many traditional dishes, including the Lamb Tagine with Glazed Cinnamon Figs (page 165). Garam masala, used in this mix, is a blend of cinnamon, nutmeg, cloves, cardamom and a pinch of saffron.

¼ cup (60 mL) sweet Spanish paprika
¼ cup (60 mL) garam masala
1 Tbsp (15 mL) ground ginger
1 Tbsp (15 mL) ground cumin
2 tsp (10 mL) ground coriander

Blend the paprika, garam masala, ginger, cumin and coriander in a small bowl. Place in a sealed container and store in a cool place for up to 6 months.

MEDITERRANEAN RUB

This chunky Mediterranean rub is excellent for coating meats such as fillet of beef, pork tenderloin or rack of lamb before roasting. Use it to make Mediterranean Rack of Lamb (page 163).

½ cup (125 mL) chopped Italian parsley

½ cup (125 mL) toasted pine nuts

¼ cup (60 mL) finely chopped shallots

3 cloves of garlic, finely chopped

1 Tbsp (15 mL) Dijon mustard

1 Tbsp (15 mL) olive oil

freshly ground pepper to taste

1 OR 2 DAYS BEFORE Combine the parsley, pine nuts, shallots, garlic, mustard, olive oil and pepper in a food processor. Process until slightly chunky. Place in a sealed container and refrigerate overnight. Will keep for 2 days.

Makes about 1¼ cups (310 mL)

PER SERVING
78 calories
1 g protein
8 g fat
5 g carbohydrate
1 g fiber
18 mg sodium

drinks and small bites

MINT TEA

A relaxing hot drink finale to a Moroccan dinner, or to enjoy any time of day. Pick up the decorative tea glasses and silver tea pot at Middle Eastern delis or gift shops for the authentic presentation.

⅓ cup (75 mL) coarsely chopped mint leaves

1 Tbsp (15 mL) white sugar

2 tsp (10 mL) or 2 tea bags green tea

2 tsp (10 mL) or 2 tea bags mint tea

3 cups (750 mL) boiling water

Place the mint, sugar and tea bags in a teapot. Pour in the boiling water. Let steep about 3 minutes for flavors to blend. Pour into glasses. Serve immediately.

Makes 6 small tea glass servings

PER SERVING
8 calories
0 g protein
0 g fat
2 g carbohydrate
0 g fiber
0 mg sodium

CRANGRIA BLANCA

Serves 8 to 12

PER SERVING
180 calories
1 g protein
0 g fat
42 g carbohydrate
1 g fiber
8 mg sodium

Sangria is wonderfully refreshing when made with white wine rather than the traditional more robust red wine. I also add Ocean Spray White Cranberry juice for a surprisingly refreshing taste. This version omits the sugar, but with the fresh fruit and lemon soda giving us the perfect balance of taste and flavor we don't need it. I like to serve Crangria Blanca during a summer evening of entertaining with a Spanish tapas platter that includes Artichoke Frittata (page 121), Roasted Almonds with Smoked Paprika (page 126), Rand's Roasted Beets with Yogurt (page 130) and Flatbreads with Greek Pressed Yogurt (page 125).

two 3 cup (750 mL) bottles of white wine, Chardonnay or Pinot Grigio

1 cup (250 mL) orange liqueur or fresh orange juice

2 cups (500 mL) Ocean Spray White Cranberry juice

3 ripe peaches or nectarines, peeled and sliced

1 lime, thinly sliced

1 orange, thinly sliced

1 lemon, thinly sliced

3 cups (750 mL) lemon soda

crushed ice

SEVERAL HOURS BEFORE SERVING Combine the wine, orange liqueur or orange juice, white cranberry juice, peaches, lime, orange and lemon. Cover and refrigerate.

JUST BEFORE SERVING Pour into a large pitcher and add the soda. Pour into wine goblets and add crushed ice.

MEXICAN ARTICHOKE BITES

Not only are these nippy appetizers low in calories, they're also my emergency favorites because they're so quick to put together at the last minute. Teenagers love them and they make great après-ski nibbles, too. Try a batch and watch them disappear.

one 12 oz (340 mL) jar marinated artichoke hearts

½ cup (125 mL) Hellman's low-fat mayonnaise

1 cup (250 mL) grated Parmesan cheese

one 4 oz (113 g) can chopped mild green chilies

dash of Tabasco sauce

one 1 lb (454 g) package flat white corn tortilla chips with zero trans fat

1 OR 2 DAYS BEFORE Drain and finely chop the artichoke hearts. Combine the artichokes with the mayonnaise, ½ cup (125 mL) Parmesan cheese, chilies and Tabasco, in a medium-sized bowl, stirring well to blend. Cover and refrigerate until ready to serve.

TO SERVE Lay out the tortilla chips in an even layer on a large baking sheet. Cover the surface of each chip with about 1 to 2 tsp (5 to 10 mL) of the mixture. Repeat until the mixture is used up.

Sprinkle with the remaining ½ cup (125 mL) of Parmesan cheese and broil until they're hot and golden. Watch carefully as they can burn quickly. Or preheat the oven to 400°F (200°C) and bake until hot, about 5 to 8 minutes. Serve immediately.

Makes about 4 dozen

PER 3-PIECE SERVING
90 calories
4 g protein
3 g fat
14 g carbohydrate
3 g fiber
200 mg sodium

BRUSCHETTA *with* RICOTTA CHEESE SPREAD

Serves 8 to 10 as an appetizer,
6 as a salad or 10 as an
antipasto

PER 1-CROSTINO SERVING
75 calories
5 g protein
3 g fat
7 g carbohydrate
2 g fiber
120 mg sodium

This is the perfect do-ahead Italian appetizer for summertime entertaining when local heirloom tomatoes are at their peak. I've substituted low-fat yogurt for the chèvre in my classic bruschetta recipe to make it a healthy choice. The ricotta cheese spread can be made 1 or 2 days ahead but the bruschetta should be prepared the day of serving.

RICOTTA CHEESE SPREAD

1 cup (250 mL) low-fat ricotta cheese

½ cup (125 mL) Pressed Yogurt (page 131)

¼ cup (60 mL) finely chopped green onions

3 Tbsp (45 mL) finely chopped basil

1 Tbsp (15 mL) Reduced Balsamic Vinegar (see sidebar)

BRUSCHETTA

2½ cups (625 mL) Roma or regular tomatoes, cut into
small chunks

½ cup (125 mL) chopped sun-dried tomatoes in olive oil
(optional)

½ cup (125 mL) finely chopped green onions

½ cup (125 mL) thin julienne strips of basil

2 to 3 cloves of garlic, finely chopped

2 Tbsp (30 mL) olive oil

1 Tbsp (15 mL) balsamic or red wine vinegar

freshly ground pepper to taste

basil leaves for garnish

Crostini (page 161)

1 OR 2 DAYS BEFORE Prepare the Ricotta Cheese Spread. Combine the ricotta cheese, Pressed Yogurt, green onions, basil and Reduced Balsamic Vinegar in a bowl. Cover and refrigerate overnight.

DAY OF SERVING Prepare the bruschetta. Discard the seeds from the chopped tomatoes and drain well. Mix everything together except the basil leaves and Crostini, and let sit covered at room temperature for several hours.

TO SERVE Strain the excess juice from the bruschetta. Spoon a mound of the cheese spread in the center of a large platter. Drizzle the Reduced Balsamic Vinegar over the cheese spread. Surround the cheese with a circle of bruschetta. Garnish the tray with the basil leaves. Serve with plenty of crostini in a basket, and let the guests top each crostini with a dollop of the cheese spread and a little of the bruschetta.

ANTIPASTO PRESENTATION Add a bowl of assorted marinated Italian olives and a platter with wedges of melon wrapped around thin slices of prosciutto.

Chef's Secret

REDUCED BALSAMIC VINEGAR To make reduced balsamic vinegar, also known as balsamic syrup, warm a frying pan over low heat. Pour in ½ cup (125 mL) balsamic vinegar plus 2 Tbsp (30 mL) brown sugar and simmer 2 to 3 minutes until they reduce to a syrup and measure about ⅓ cup (75 mL). Cool. Put in a sealed jar and refrigerate for up to 2 to 3 weeks. Some specialty shops carry an Italian balsamic syrup called balsamic cream (*crema di balsamico*), which is superb and saves time making your own. Use it to drizzle over salad plates, strawberries or figs.

ROASTED RED PEPPER HUMMUS

Makes about 2½ cups (625 mL)

PER SERVING OF 3
SMALL TRIANGLES
OF PITA BREAD

240 calories

2 g protein

22 g fat

9 g carbohydrate

4 g fiber

125 mg sodium

Hummus is a popular Mediterranean dip of cooked chickpeas (garbanzo beans) that are puréed and then blended to the consistency of thick mayonnaise. I've added roasted red peppers for a twist of flavors. Hummus is available at most delis and specialty shops, but it's fun to make your own. Serve with cucumber tzatziki and warmed pita bread.

one 14 oz (398 mL) can chickpeas
⅓ cup (75 mL) roasted red peppers (page 107)
¼ cup (60 mL) lemon juice
¼ cup (60 mL) tahini (sesame paste)
1 clove of garlic, finely chopped
½ tsp (2 mL) cumin
freshly ground pepper to taste
½ to ¾ cup (125 to 175 mL) olive oil

1 OR 2 DAYS BEFORE Drain the chickpeas and rinse them with cold water. Purée everything but the olive oil in a blender or food processor. Gradually add ½ cup (125 mL) of the oil. If the mixture seems dry, add the remaining oil until the hummus is creamy like a dip. Cover and refrigerate.

TO SERVE Moisten with more olive oil and lemon juice if the hummus seems too dry.

ARTICHOKE FRITTATA

This appetizer always brings raves. A frittata is similar to a quiche but doesn't have the crust. Goes well with an antipasto or tapas menu, or on its own!

one 12 oz (340 mL) jar, plus one 6 oz (175 mL) jar marinated artichokes (about 2 cups/500 mL total)

1 cup (250 mL) grated low-fat cheddar cheese or Spanish Manchego cheese, plus 2 to 3 Tbsp (30 to 45 mL) more for garnish

⅓ cup (75 mL) finely chopped green onions

⅓ cup (75 mL) chopped sun-dried tomatoes in oil

¼ cup (60 mL) crushed unsalted crackers (about 6)

2 Tbsp (30 mL) drained and chopped roasted red pepper

3 large eggs, lightly beaten

dash of Tabasco sauce

freshly ground pepper to taste

1 OR 2 DAYS BEFORE Preheat the oven to 325°F (160°C). Lightly grease an 8-inch (20 cm) or 9-inch (22 cm) quiche pan with vegetable oil. Drain the artichokes and chop them into small pieces. Mix in a large bowl with the 1 cup (250 mL) of cheese, green onions, sun-dried tomatoes, crackers, roasted pepper, eggs, Tabasco and pepper. Pour into the prepared pan. Sprinkle the remaining cheese on top. Bake 30 to 35 minutes until golden and a knife inserted into the center comes out clean. Cool, cover and refrigerate.

TO SERVE Cover and reheat in a 350°F (180°C) about 20 minutes, or until warmed. Cut into 1½ inch (3.5 cm) squares and serve. Slices will be thin. You can also freeze the squares after baking. Just thaw overnight and reheat.

Serves 8

PER SERVING
155 calories
14 g protein
7 g fat
11 g carbohydrate
4 g fiber
280 mg sodium

Chef's Secret
MANCHEGO CHEESE
Manchego cheese from Spain is found at most cheese delis and is superb in this frittata because of its sharp taste. If unavailable, low-fat cheddar cheese will be fine.

ITALIAN PIZZATA BITES

*Makes 16 pizzata wedges,
enough to serve 4 as an
appetizer or to accompany
soups and salads*

PER PIECE

59 calories
5 g protein
2 g fat
7 g carbohydrate
1 g fiber
200 mg sodium

Everyone loves these fun-to-make mini pizza appetizer bites, which are not only tasty but also nutritious. As Doug always comments, "Delish and nutrish." The secret is using whole wheat pita wraps for the crust. Pick up bottled tapenades, antipasto and caramelized onions from your local deli or let your imagination go wild, using condiments and fresh vegetables that you have on hand. Add a hearty tossed green salad and you have an easy weekday dinner.

two 6-inch (15 cm) whole wheat pita wraps

TAPENADE, CHEESE, TOMATO AND PROSCIUTTO TOPPINGS

¼ cup (60 mL) sun-dried tomato or olive tapenade, or other deli choices

½ cup (125 mL) thinly sliced cherry tomatoes

¼ cup (60 mL) mini bocconcini balls, cut into 3 slices each, or ¼ cup (60 mL) grated pecorino or Parmesan cheese

¼ lb (125 g) thinly sliced prosciutto, coarsely chopped

3 Tbsp (45 mL) chopped basil

SEVERAL HOURS BEFORE SERVING Put the 2 pita wraps on a large plate. Spread half of the toppings evenly on each, starting with the tapenade. Top with the tomatoes and bocconcini overlapping. Sprinkle with prosciutto. Cover and refrigerate.

TO SERVE Preheat the oven to 400°F (200°C). Place the pizzatas on a baking sheet or pizza pan. Bake 8 to 10 minutes until the cheese is melted and the pizzatas are crispy. Sprinkle with basil. Slice each pita wrap into 8 triangle wedges and serve.

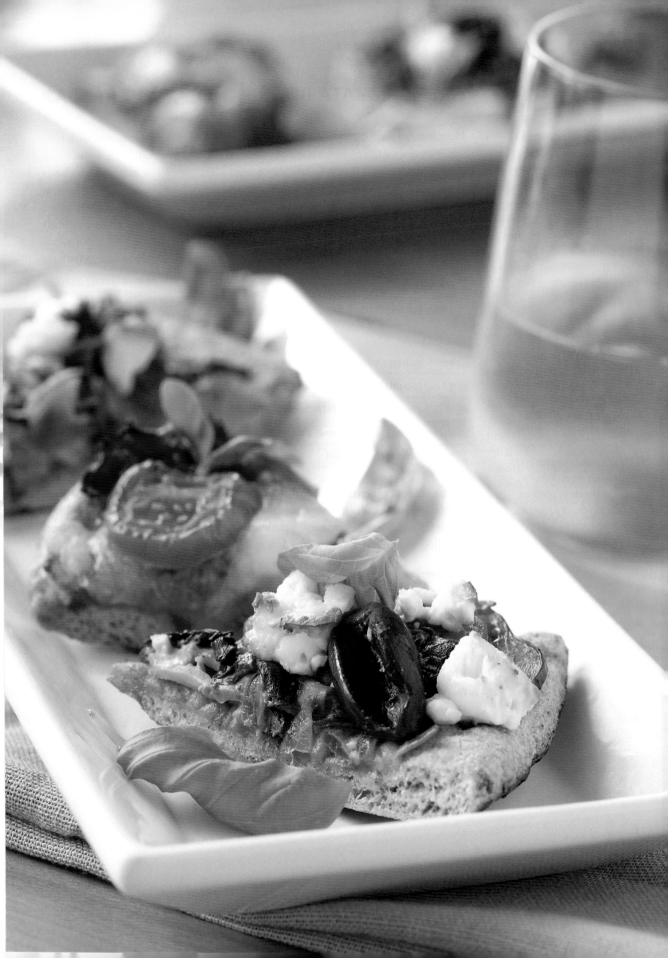

ROASTED ALMONDS *with* SMOKED PAPRIKA

Makes 3 cups (750 mL)
(about 12 dozen)

PER SERVING OF 12
ALMONDS
181 calories
7 g protein
16 g fat
5 g carbohydrate
4 g fiber
580 mg sodium

Chef's Secret

THE ORIGIN OF TAPAS
Centuries ago, when
horsemen traveled from
town to town, hungry and
thirsty, tavern keepers
prepared glasses of wine
and sherry and covered
them with a tapa, or lid,
made of slices of ham,
cheese or bread to protect
the wine from dust, flies
and rain.

The Spanish Marcona almonds are the best in the world, and are served at every tapas bar throughout Spain. They're hard to find in North America, but if you locate them, use them for this recipe. The teaser taste is the combination of ground smoked sweet paprika and sea salt. Make 4 to 5 days ahead for the flavors to marry. They keep for weeks and are great for emergency entertaining. A Spanish sherry is a perfect partner for these nuts.

3 cups (750 mL) whole blanched almonds

2½ tsp (12 mL) celery seeds (optional)

1 Tbsp (15 mL) sea salt

2½ tsp (12 mL) La Chinata smoked sweet paprika

1 Tbsp (15 mL) olive oil

4 OR 5 DAYS BEFORE Preheat the oven to 350°F (180°C). Place the almonds on a large baking sheet. Roast 10 minutes, tossing occasionally to ensure even roasting. Reduce the temperature to 325°F (160°C) and roast about 8 to 10 minutes longer, or until golden.

Meanwhile, roast the celery seeds (if using) in a small frying pan over low heat about 2 minutes. Grind the salt and the celery seeds in a coffee grinder to a powder as fine as icing sugar. Combine the paprika, celery seeds and salt in a small bowl, blending well. Set aside.

When the nuts are golden, put into a large mixing bowl. Drizzle with the olive oil and toss to coat evenly. Add the paprika and celery seed mixture, tossing well. Return to the baking sheet and roast about 3 to 4 minutes longer. Cool. Store in an airtight container for up to 1 month.

MUSHROOMS *with* GARLIC

Every Spanish tapas bar serves a plate of sautéed mushrooms. I like to use a variety of mushrooms for flavor and texture. Have a basket of rustic bread to soak up the juices. Prepare just before your guests arrive, reheat a few minutes and serve.

Serves 6

PER SERVING
335 calories
9 g protein
9 g fat
66 g carbohydrate
10 g fiber
15 mg sodium

2 Tbsp (30 mL) olive oil

1 lb (500 g) mixed stemmed mushrooms, crimini, shiitake, oyster and chanterelle, cut in large pieces

4 cloves of garlic, finely chopped

3 Tbsp (45 mL) dry sherry (fino)

juice of ½ lemon

freshly ground pepper to taste

pinch of red pepper flakes

⅓ cup (75 mL) toasted pine nuts (see sidebar page 128)

3 Tbsp (45 mL) finely chopped Italian parsley

JUST BEFORE SERVING Warm the olive oil in a large frying pan over medium heat. Sauté the mushrooms until they start to soften, about 2 minutes. Add the garlic and sauté until softened and most of the liquid has evaporated, about 3 minutes. Add the sherry, lemon juice, pepper and red pepper flakes.

TO SERVE Put into a serving dish and sprinkle with the pine nuts and parsley. Serve while hot.

FETA CHEESE *with* LEMON ZEST, PINE NUTS *and* OLIVES

Serves 6 to 8

....

PER SERVING
432 calories
16 g protein
34 g fat
34 g carbohydrate
4 g fiber
1280 mg sodium

Chef's Secret
TOASTED PINE NUTS

Preheat the oven to 350°F (180°C). Spread the nuts on a single layer on a baking sheet. Roast about 4 to 5 minutes, or just until golden. Watch that they don't burn, as they'll taste bitter. Store in a sealed container for 2 months. Add toasted pine nuts to salads for a nutritious crunch.

I like to serve this starter cheese dish on its own or add it to an antipasto or tapas platter. Serve with warmed pita bread or Pita Crisps (page 159).

MARINADE

3 Tbsp (45 mL) olive oil

2 Tbsp (30 mL) chopped fresh basil

2 Tbsp (30 mL) chopped fresh oregano

2 Tbsp (30 mL) lemon juice

1 Tbsp (15 mL) lemon zest

1 Tbsp (15 mL) finely chopped fresh rosemary

freshly ground pepper to taste

¾ lb (375 g) sheep or goat feta cheese

¼ cup (60 mL) toasted pine nuts

⅓ cup (75 mL) kalamata olives, pitted, sliced in half

⅓ cup (75 mL) Greek green olives, pitted and sliced in half, or quartered if large

A FEW HOURS BEFORE Whisk together the olive oil, basil, oregano, lemon juice and zest, rosemary and pepper in a small bowl. Cover and refrigerate.

TO SERVE Arrange the cheese on a platter. Drizzle the marinade over the cheese. Top with the pine nuts and olives. Serve with the Pita Crisps or warmed pita bread.

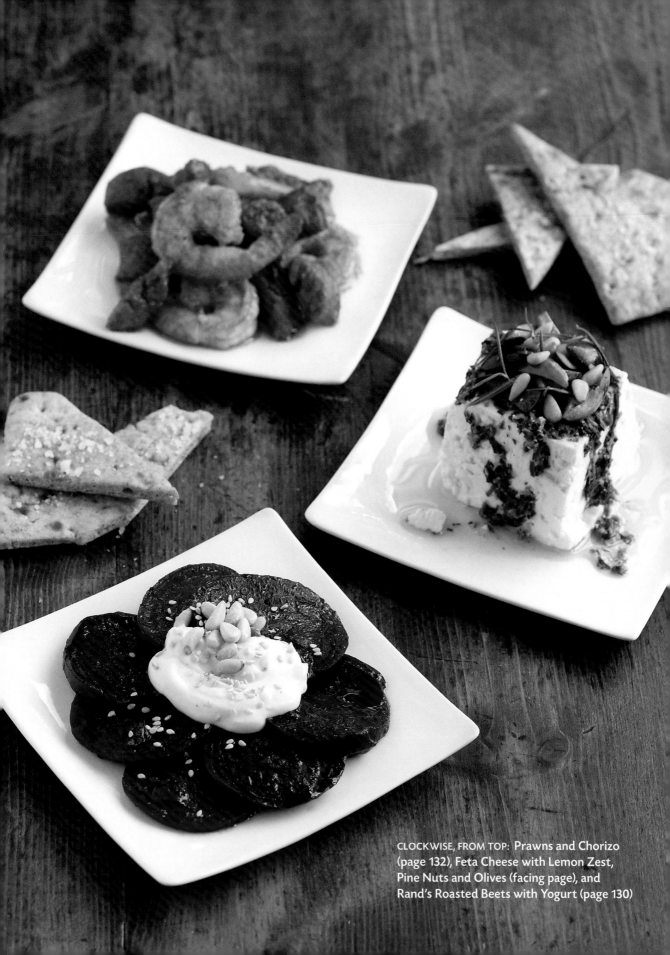

CLOCKWISE, FROM TOP: Prawns and Chorizo
(page 132), Feta Cheese with Lemon Zest,
Pine Nuts and Olives (facing page), and
Rand's Roasted Beets with Yogurt (page 130)

RAND'S ROASTED BEETS *with* YOGURT

Serves 6 to 8

PER SERVING
231 calories
8 g protein
16 g fat
15 g carbohydrate
3 g fiber
88 mg sodium

Our son, Rand, loves beets, so I always include this colorful, tasty addition to my Moroccan salads (see the Taste of Morocco menu on page 56), Italian antipasto platter or Spanish tapas. Serve with flatbreads.

LEMON PARSLEY VINAIGRETTE

¼ cup (125 mL) lemon juice

3 Tbsp (45 mL) finely chopped Italian parsley

1 clove of garlic, finely chopped

½ cup (125 mL) olive oil

freshly ground pepper to taste

ROASTED BEETS

2 lbs (1 kg) beets (about 8 large)

1 Tbsp (15 mL) olive oil

2 Tbsp (30 mL) toasted pine nuts for garnish (see sidebar page 128)

2 Tbsp (30 mL) toasted sesame seeds for garnish (page 97)

GREEK YOGURT SPREAD

1 cup (250 mL) Pressed Yogurt (see facing page)

1 Tbsp (15 mL) red wine vinegar or sherry vinegar

2 cloves of garlic, finely chopped

½ tsp (2 mL) Spanish smoked sweet paprika (optional)

freshly ground pepper to taste

1 OR 2 DAYS BEFORE Prepare the Lemon Parsley Vinaigrette. In a small bowl, whisk together the lemon juice, parsley and garlic while slowly adding the olive oil. Add pepper to taste. Store in a sealed jar in the refrigerator.

Cook the beets. Preheat the oven to 425°F (220°C). Cut off the beet roots, and wash and wipe dry. Slice each beet in half from top to bottom. Wrap individually in aluminum foil and place on a baking sheet. Roast about 1 hour or until tender. Check by sticking a knife into the beets to make sure they're cooked. Alternatively, boil the beets in water to cover, about 25 to 30 minutes, or until they're cooked. Cool, peel, thinly slice and put into a bowl. Add enough Lemon Parsley Vinaigrette to coat the cooked beets well. Cover and refrigerate.

THE DAY BEFORE Prepare the Greek Yogurt Spread.

Blend the Pressed Yogurt, vinegar, garlic, paprika (if using), and pepper in a small bowl. Cover and refrigerate overnight.

SEVERAL HOURS BEFORE SERVING Arrange the beet slices on a platter. Spoon the Greek yogurt mixture over the beets and swirl the yogurt to cover the beets. Drizzle a little olive oil over the beets and yogurt. Cover and refrigerate until ready to serve.

JUST BEFORE SERVING Sprinkle with toasted pine nuts and toasted sesame seeds. Serve with flatbreads.

PRESSED YOGURT *Makes about 1 cup (250 mL)*

An ideal alternative to high-fat sour cream or whipping cream for dips, sauces, salad dressings and toppings for soups, vegetables and fruits. Commercial yogurt strainers are excellent, and are available in most kitchen shops. A coffee filter or cheesecloth placed over a glass bowl also works well.

2 cups (500 mL) low-fat plain yogurt

1 OR 2 DAYS BEFORE Spoon the yogurt into a strainer, coffee filter or cheesecloth placed over a bowl. Cover with plastic wrap, and refrigerate for a few hours for a slightly thickened yogurt cheese, or overnight for a thick spreading cheese consistency. Store in a covered jar in the refrigerator. Will keep for 1 week.

PRAWNS *and* CHORIZO

Serves 6

PER SERVING
230 calories
28 g protein
11 g fat
1 g carbohydrate
0 g fiber
285 mg sodium

Another classic tapas dish with a dynamic presentation served throughout Spain. The chorizo sausage gives the prawns a jolt. I allow about 4 to 5 prawns per person as part of a tapas platter.

3 Tbsp (45 mL) olive oil

½ lb (250 g) cured mild smoked or unsmoked chorizo sausage, cut into small cubes

4 cloves of garlic, finely chopped

½ tsp (2 mL) smoked sweet paprika

24 to 30 large uncooked peeled prawns, tails left on

3 Tbsp (45 mL) dry sherry (fino)

JUST BEFORE SERVING Warm the oil in a frying pan over medium heat. Add the chorizo and sauté a few minutes until crisp. Add the garlic and smoked paprika. Sauté 1 or 2 minutes until the garlic is softened. Add the prawns and sherry and sauté until opaque, 2 to 3 minutes.

TO SERVE Put into an attractive medium-sized serving bowl to take to the table. Serve with plenty of rustic bread to soak up the juices.

TUNA *and* OLIVE TAPENADE PÂTÉ

Take a can of tuna and a container of olive tapenade from the deli and you have the makings for a quick, tasty appetizer. Serve with Pita Crisps (page 159) or Crostini (page 161).

one 6 oz (175 g) can low-sodium light tuna, in oil, drained

¼ cup (60 mL) green or black olive tapenade

2 tsp (10 mL) Dijon mustard

3 Tbsp (45 mL) lemon juice

freshly ground pepper to taste

Combine the tuna, olive tapenade, mustard, lemon juice and pepper in a food processor and process until creamy and smooth. If needed, add a little more olive tapenade and lemon juice to make it very creamy.

Makes about 1 cup (250 mL), enough to serve 4 to 6

PER 1 TBSP (15 ML) SERVING
39 calories
5 g protein
2 g fat
1 g carbohydrate
0 g fiber
120 mg sodium

GLAZED FRESH FIGS *in* BALSAMIC *with* CHÈVRE

Serves 6

....

PER SERVING
157 calories
20 g protein
0 g fat
20 g carbohydrate
1 g fiber
1500 mg sodium

Chef's Secret

SURPRISE ATTRACTION
Add ½ lb (250 g) fresh strawberries, stemmed and sliced in half. Glaze the strawberries with ⅓ cup (75 mL) warm Reduced Balsamic Vinegar. Cool. Serve with figs and cheese.

Pick up some specialty thin fruit crackers to complement the figs and cheese toppings. Black figs are the best.

⅓ cup (75 mL) Reduced Balsamic Vinegar (page 118)
....
6 fresh figs cut in half from top to bottom
....
1½ cups (375 mL) chèvre (goat cheese), sheep feta or Spanish
    Manchego cheese, or a combination of all 3 cheeses

ON THE DAY OF SERVING Warm the Reduced Balsamic Vinegar in a frying pan over low heat. Add the figs, turning with tongs to glaze evenly. Cool.

TO SERVE Slice the figs in half again. Put on a platter with the cheese and drizzle any leftover Reduced Balsamic Vinegar over the figs. Let guests help themselves to a wedge of cheese topping the fig.

GUACAMOLE

This is my new healthy version of the classic guacamole, and our family's request every time I serve Mexican food or feel in the mood for guacamole and corn chips. It's half the calories and half the fat of my original family recipe. By replacing high-fat sour cream with low-fat sour cream, we can indulge in Guacamole and chips without the guilt! Just don't go overboard with the chips. Lime juice instead of lemon juice is the teaser citrus taste.

5 large ripe avocados

1 cup (250 mL) low-fat sour cream

½ cup (125 mL) chopped peeled tomatoes

¼ cup (60 mL) finely chopped green onions

¼ cup (125 mL) lime juice

2 Tbsp (30 mL) Tomato and Red Onion Salsa (page 110, optional)

1 Tbsp (15 mL) white wine vinegar

2 tsp (10 mL) chili powder, or to taste

1 tsp (5 mL) ground cumin or 1 Tbsp (15 mL) Tex-Mex Seasoning (page 177)

freshly ground pepper to taste

Tex-Max Salmon Tacos (page 177)

unsalted corn chips

ABOUT 1 HOUR BEFORE SERVING Peel the avocados and remove the pits. Place in a medium-sized bowl, and mash until slightly chunky. Set aside 1 avocado pit and ½ cup (125 mL) of the sour cream. Combine the remaining sour cream, tomatoes, green onions, lime juice, salsa (if using), vinegar, chili powder, cumin and pepper and mix well. Add the avocado pit (to prevent the avocados from darkening) and spread the reserved sour cream in a thin layer to cover the guacamole mixture. Cover and refrigerate.

JUST BEFORE SERVING Remove the avocado pit and fold in the sour cream topping. Adjust the seasonings to taste.

TO SERVE Serve with the Tex-Mex Salmon Tacos, along with a basket of the corn chips for dipping. Or try it with your favorite Mexican dish.

Makes about 3 cups (750 mL), enough to serve 8 to 10

PER SERVING
250 calories
4 g protein
18 g fat
19 g carbohydrate
5 g fiber
140 mg sodium

CHICKEN SATAY *with* SPICY PEANUT DIP

Serves 6 to 8

PER SERVING OF 4 PIECES

320 calories

32 g protein

15 g fat

11 g carbohydrate

1 g fiber

375 mg sodium

This classic appetizer has been a winning opener to many parties at our home for over 3 decades. However, with coconut milk as the base for the original Spicy Peanut Dip, I was faced with a dilemma—the fat content sky rocketed when we did the nutritional analysis. Low-fat yogurt came to my rescue, making this satay a healthy treat. This is also the perfect choice to complement the Asian Express menu (page 57).

SPICY PEANUT DIP

1 cup (250 mL) chunky peanut butter

1 to 1½ cups (250 to 375 mL) low-fat plain yogurt

3 Tbsp (45 mL) lemon juice

2 Tbsp (30 mL) toasted sesame seeds (page 97)

2 Tbsp (30 mL) light soy sauce

2 Tbsp (30 mL) sesame oil

1 Tbsp (15 mL) Chinese sweet chili sauce

1 Tbsp (15 mL) brown sugar

2 cloves of garlic, finely chopped

2 tsp (10 mL) lemon zest

CHICKEN SATAY

½ cup (125 mL) sake

¼ cup (60 mL) sesame oil

¼ cup (60 mL) light soy sauce

8 boneless and skinless chicken breasts

small 5-inch (12 cm) wooden skewers

24 to 30 asparagus spears (allowing 4 to 5 per person)

1 OR 2 DAYS BEFORE Prepare the Spicy Peanut Dip. Combine the peanut butter, 1 cup (250 mL) yogurt, lemon juice, sesame seeds, soy sauce, sesame oil, chili sauce, sugar, garlic and zest in a food processor. Blend just until smooth. Slowly add the remaining ½ cup (125 mL) of yogurt so that the mixture is just thick enough for dipping the chicken and asparagus.

DAY OF SERVING Prepare the Chicken Satay. Combine the sake, sesame oil and soy sauce in a large bowl. Add the chicken, cover and refrigerate for 2 to 3 hours to marinate. Preheat the oven to 350°F (180°C). Remove the chicken from the marinade and place on a large baking sheet. Bake about 30 to 35 minutes, or until tender but without pink juices. Cool, then cut into 1-inch (2.5 cm) cubes, cover and refrigerate.

TO SERVE Bring the peanut dip to room temperature and thin with a little more yogurt if necessary. Place 1 chicken cube on each small skewer and fan them out on a large platter with the peanut sauce in the center for dipping. Decorate the platter with an exotic flower.

Chef's Secret

ASPARAGUS WITH SPICY PEANUT DIP For vegetarians, substitute asparagus spears for chicken, allowing 4 to 5 asparagus spears per person. The day before, trim and clean 24 to 30 asparagus spears. Blanch for 2 to 3 minutes in a large saucepan with about 1 inch (2.5 cm) of boiling water, until just tender-crisp, about 2 to 3 minutes. Don't overcook. Drain and chill in ice water. Pat dry and layer between paper towels on a large plate. Cover and refrigerate until ready to serve. To serve, arrange the asparagus on a separate platter with a bowl of the satay dip in the middle.

PER SERVING
OF 4 OR 5 PIECES
280 calories
7 g protein
23 g fat
15 g carbohydrate
3 g fiber
360 mg sodium

full of vitamins

Vegetables

VEGETABLE GRATIN

Here's a quick "emergency" vegetable dish that my family just loves. It's low in fat, high in taste and provides your entire vegetable plate all in 1 dish. Make it ahead of time for a small or large crowd; it's easy to multiply. Add a roasted chicken to complement the vegetables, such as Marietta's Italian Roasted Chicken (page 172), and your dinner is all set. And for vegetarians, it's a winner all on its own.

10 small red or white new potatoes, thinly sliced
2 small zucchini thinly sliced
7 Roma tomatoes, thinly sliced
6 Tbsp (90 mL) grated Parmesan cheese
⅓ cup (75 mL) chopped basil leaves, packed
½ tsp (2 mL) dried thyme
½ tsp (2 mL) dried oregano
olive oil for drizzling
⅓ cup (75 mL) low-sodium chicken or vegetable stock

Serves 6

PER SERVING
250 calories
9 g protein
2 g fat
51 g carbohydrate
6 g fiber
100 mg sodium

SEVERAL HOURS BEFORE SERVING Lightly grease a shallow 13- by 9-inch (3.5 L) casserole dish with vegetable oil. Line the casserole with a layer of half of the potato slices, half the zucchini slices and half the tomato slices. Sprinkle on half the cheese, basil, thyme and oregano evenly, and drizzle a little olive oil over all. Layer the remaining potatoes, zucchini and tomatoes, and sprinkle the remaining cheese and herbs over all. Pour the chicken stock evenly over the vegetables. Cover and refrigerate until ready to bake.

2 HOURS BEFORE SERVING Take the casserole out of the refrigerator and preheat the oven to 400°F (200°C). Bake 40 to 45 minutes or until the potatoes are tender.

ROASTED VEGETABLES

Serves 6

PER SERVING
250 calories
5 g protein
5 g fat
50 g carbohydrate
7 g fiber
100 mg sodium

Chef's Secret

RICH MIXTURE: HERBES DE PROVENCE Herbes de Provence is a herb mixture used in many French dishes, and varies according to the chef's dish. It's usually an equal blend of dried oregano, thyme, marjoram, savory and rosemary, and sometimes culinary lavender. You can find it in specialty shops or make your own. Dried culinary lavender is hard to find and is not included in all herbes de Provence.

Roasted vegetables go with everything, from a festive turkey to barbecued steak. Try this combination of vegetables or include parsnips, turnips and sliced fennel. For quantities, allow 1 or 2 pieces of each vegetable per person. You can prepare the vegetables a day ahead, but they're best made the day of serving. Prep them in the morning and then set aside on baking sheets until ready to roast.

12 unpeeled small new baby potatoes

3 large yams, peeled and cut into twelve 1-inch (2.5 cm) cubes

4 large beets, peeled and cut into twelve 1-inch (2.5 cm) cubes

3 medium-sized carrots, peeled and cut into twelve 1-inch (2.5 cm) cubes

3 Tbsp (45 mL) olive oil

3 Tbsp (45 mL) finely chopped rosemary or 1 Tbsp (15 mL) herbes de Provence

Preheat the oven to 350°F (180°C) and lightly grease 2 large baking sheets with olive oil. Place the 4 vegetables in separate bowls. Toss each with enough of the olive oil just to coat, and sprinkle each with the rosemary or herbes de Provence. Place the new potatoes and yams on 1 baking sheet and the beets and carrots on the remaining baking sheet, spreading them out in a single layer to roast evenly.

Roast uncovered about 25 minutes. Toss and brush with a little more of the oil if needed. Roast about 25 minutes longer or until the vegetables are cooked. Check the vegetables often during the last 10 minutes of cooking because some vegetables roast faster than others (beets take the longest). Remove the cooked vegetables from the oven as they are done and set them aside in a serving dish. Toss all the vegetables together once they're roasted, adding the beets just before serving so they won't color the other vegetables.

TO SERVE Serve immediately. If roasted ahead, preheat the oven to 350°F (180°C) and reheat the vegetables, uncovered, about 25 minutes or until warmed.

GREEN BEANS *with* SHIITAKE MUSHROOMS

This vegetable duo takes green beans to a new level with the addition of the exquisite taste of shiitake mushrooms. It has now become a tradition to include it as one of the star vegetable dishes for our Thanksgiving or Christmas dinner menu.

2 Tbsp (30 mL) unsalted butter
½ lb (250 g) shiitake mushrooms, stemmed and sliced
⅓ cup (75 mL) chopped shallots
3 cloves of garlic, finely chopped
2 lb (1 kg) thin green beans, trimmed
⅔ cup (150 mL) low-sodium chicken broth
freshly ground pepper to taste

Serves 8 to 10

PER SERVING
165 calories
5 g protein
4 g fat
28 g carbohydrate
6 g fiber
11 mg sodium

THE DAY BEFORE Melt 1 Tbsp (15 mL) of the butter in a large frying pan. Add the mushrooms and sauté until softened, about 3 minutes. Set aside. Melt the remaining 1 Tbsp (15 mL) butter in the same frying pan. Add the shallots and the garlic and sauté until softened, about 2 minutes. Add the green beans and toss to coat. Add the chicken broth. Cover and simmer until the liquid evaporates and the green beans are still slightly crisp, about 6 to 8 minutes. Add the sautéed mushrooms and toss well. Season with the pepper. Put them in a shallow 13- by 9-inch (3.5 L) casserole dish. Cover and refrigerate.

TO SERVE Preheat the oven to 350°F (180°C). Cover the beans and reheat for 20 to 25 minutes or until warmed.

YAM *and* BUTTERNUT SQUASH PURÉE

Serves 6 to 8

....

PER SERVING
394 calories
6 g protein
4 g fat
85 g carbohydrate
10 g fiber
25 mg sodium

Chef's Secret
VEGGIE TRIO VARIATION
Add 1 cup (250 mL) sliced
cooked carrots or parsnips
for a vegetable trio purée.
Add the cooked carrots
or parsnips to the food
processor along with
the yams and butternut
squash. It will take a little
longer to purée when
adding cooked carrots.

Purées of vegetables are always a big hit as a side vegetable dish. Yams are full of vitamins A and C, fiber, potassium and calcium, making them one of the most nutritionally sound vegetables. This combination of yams and butternut squash is like velvet. It's another family choice to complement a festive turkey.

4 lb (2 kg) yams, washed, sliced lengthwise
2 lb (1 kg) butternut squash, washed, halved and seeded
⅓ cup (75 mL) orange juice
1 tsp (5 mL) freshly ground pepper
¼ tsp (1 mL) freshly grated nutmeg or ground nutmeg
⅓ cup (75 mL) chopped toasted pecans (optional)

1 OR 2 DAYS BEFORE Preheat the oven to 400°F (200°C) and lightly grease 1 or 2 large baking sheets with vegetable oil. Place the yams and the squash halves cut side down on the prepared baking sheet. Roast about 1 hour until both vegetables are soft. Check by piercing with a knife after 45 minutes. When cooked, cool and peel, discarding the skin. Cut the yams and squash into large chunks and place in a food processor. Add the orange juice, pepper and nutmeg and purée until very creamy. Spoon into a 13- by 9-inch (3.5-L) casserole dish that you've lightly greased with vegetable oil.

TO SERVE Preheat the oven to 350°F (180°C). Cover with aluminum foil and reheat about 35 to 40 minutes or until heated through. Top with the nuts if desired and serve.

OVEN FRENCH FRIES

No guilt in enjoying a treat of French fries! Oven roasting, rather than deep frying in fat, is the secret. Slice the potatoes ahead of time, keep them in ice water, then pat dry and bake just before serving. They're great for dipping into Quick Lemon Dill Mayonnaise (page 108), Roasted Garlic Aioli (page 109), or simply low-fat Hellman's mayonnaise and ketchup. Try making oven fries with yams. They roast faster, in about 15 minutes.

6 large baking potatoes (Yukon Gold or Idaho) or yams

vegetable oil

½ cup (125 mL) finely grated Parmesan (optional)

Peel the potatoes and cut into French fry slices, the length of the potato. Don't make them too thin. Keep in ice water until needed.

JUST BEFORE SERVING Preheat the oven to 425°F (220°C) and lightly oil a baking sheet and a cake rack that fits on top of the baking sheet. Drain the potatoes and pat them dry. Roll them in a little oil just to coat and toss in the Parmesan cheese (if using). Place them on the cake rack on the prepared baking sheet, spreading the potatoes evenly. Bake about 50 to 55 minutes, tossing from time to time. For the last 10 minutes, remove the cake rack and spread the fries on the baking sheet to crisp. Serve immediately and watch them disappear!

Serves 6

PER SERVING
230 calories
10 g protein
5 g fat
37 g carbohydrate
4 g fiber
272 mg sodium

ROASTED ASPARAGUS

Serves 6

....

PER SERVING
100 calories
5 g protein
5 g fat
10 g carbohydrate
5 g fiber
5 mg sodium

Quick to prepare, Roasted Asparagus is an easy vegetable side dish. Combine the asparagus with Roasted Tomatoes (facing page) as a colorful and nutritious vegetable duo. I love the combination with risotto dishes, poultry and meats. Prepare ahead and roast just before serving. Cut back on the amount of asparagus depending on how many people you're serving. Roast smaller quantities in a small casserole dish rather than on a baking sheet.

3 lb (1.5 kg) asparagus spears, left whole or sliced into 3-inch (8 cm) lengths (about 3 cups/750 mL asparagus slices)
1 to 2 Tbsp (15 to 30 mL) olive oil
freshly ground pepper to taste
3 Tbsp (45 ml) lemon juice
1 Tbsp (15 mL) lemon zest

Preheat the oven to 400°F (200°C). Toss the asparagus with the olive oil, just to coat. Place on a baking sheet and sprinkle with the pepper. Roast about 10 minutes, until still crisp. Toss with the lemon juice and zest and serve.

Chef's Secret

BUYING ASPARAGUS Thin asparagus stocks are less tender, their skin more dense. Look for thicker stocks. To store until ready to use, trim the stem about ⅛ inch (3 mm) and wrap a wet paper towel around the ends to keep them fresh in the refrigerator. Before using asparagus, wash them well and snap off the tough stems.

ROASTED TOMATOES

Roasted tomatoes are my lifesavers. They make a quick side vegetable dish, and they're great for tossing into cooked pasta with added Parmesan or to complement egg dishes. Once the market farmers harvest their bright yellow cherry tomatoes, add them to your red variety. Prepare the tomato dish ahead of time, but roast just before serving.

1 lb (500 g) small tomatoes on the vine or 3 cups (750 mL) cherry tomatoes

1 to 2 Tbsp (15 to 30 mL) olive oil

freshly ground pepper to taste

Preheat the oven to 400°F (200°C). Place the tomatoes and olive oil in a bowl and toss just to coat. Place on a baking sheet and sprinkle with the pepper. Roast about 15 minutes or until they start to burst. Serve.

Serves 6

PER SERVING
69 calories
1 g protein
6 g fat
4 g carbohydrate
1 g fiber
61 mg sodium

Chef's Secret
A TOUCH OF PROVENCE
Try adding a little freshly chopped basil and a few niçoise olives to the warmed Roasted Tomatoes just before serving for a touch or Provence. *C'est si bon.*

POTATOES GRATIN

Serves 8 to 10

....

PER SERVING
266 calories
13 g protein
12 g fat
25 g carbohydrate
3 g fiber
284 mg sodium

Chef's Secret

SWEET FENNEL Fennel
is like licorice-flavored
celery. The fronds on top
of the fennel are used as
dill in salads. Fennel bulbs
are delicious baked as a
gratin or served with roast
vegetables.

No one will miss the heavy cream and butter in this lighter version of the
classic French Potatoes Gratin. Yukon Gold potatoes are the best variety
for a superb gratin. Use a mandolin for slicing the potatoes, quick and easy.
The gratin can be baked a day ahead of time and reheated just before serving.
Including the shallots, fennel and garlic adds a jolt of flavor and texture to
this gratin. It's a perfect complement to roast chicken and turkey.

2 Tbsp (30 mL) olive oil
1 cup (250 mL) finely sliced shallots or onions
1 cup (250 mL) thin julienne strips of fennel (optional)
2 cloves of garlic, finely chopped
6 cups (1.5 L) peeled, very thinly sliced Yukon Gold potatoes
freshly ground pepper to taste
1½ cups (375 mL) low-sodium chicken stock
1 cup (250 mL) skim milk
1 cup (250 mL) grated Emmenthal or Gruyère cheese
⅓ cup (75 mL) grated Parmesan cheese

Preheat the oven to 350°F (180°C). Lightly grease a 13- by 9-inch (3.5 L)
casserole dish with vegetable oil. Warm the olive oil in a frying pan over
medium heat. Add the shallots, fennel (if using) and garlic. Sauté about 3 to
4 minutes, or until softened. Set aside. Put the potatoes in a large bowl. Add
the onion and garlic mixture and the pepper. Toss well. In a separate bowl,
blend the chicken stock, skim milk and cheese. Add to the potato mixture
and mix well. Pour into the prepared casserole, pressing the potatoes down to
coat well. Add a little more chicken stock, if needed, to cover the top layer of
potatoes. Sprinkle the Parmesan cheese on top. Bake about 1½ hours, or until
the top is golden and the potatoes are cooked. Cool, cover and refrigerate.

TO SERVE Take out of the refrigerator at least 1 hour before reheating. Preheat
the oven to 350°F (180°C) and cover the casserole with aluminum foil. Reheat
about 25 to 30 minutes. Remove the foil and heat another 10 to 15 minutes or
until hot and bubbly. Serve.

fuel foods

Pasta, Rice, Beans and Bread

....

COUSCOUS *with* CHICKPEAS

Serves 10 to 12

PER SERVING
130 calories
5 g protein
1 g fat
24 g carbohydrate
4 g fiber
155 mg sodium

Couscous is a cereal from North Africa made from coarsely ground durum wheat (seminola). Use the instant variety; it works very well. Or substitute the Middle Eastern type of couscous which is a toasted variety, larger than the more familiar small-grained couscous. When cooked it swells to over double its size.

3¼ cups (810 mL) low-sodium chicken stock

3 cups (750 mL) instant couscous, regular or whole wheat

one 14 oz (398 mL) can chickpeas, drained

½ cup (125 mL) raisins or dried currants

1 tsp (5 mL) cinnamon

pinch of turmeric

2 to 3 Tbsp (30 to 45 mL) chopped Italian parsley

Bring the chicken stock to a boil in a large saucepan. Add the couscous, raisins, chickpeas, cinnamon and turmeric. Cover and let stand about 5 minutes, or until all the liquid has been absorbed. Add the parsley just before serving. Serve immediately, or cool, cover and refrigerate.

TO REHEAT Preheat the oven to 350°F (180°C) and reheat, covered, about 35 to 40 minutes or until hot. You might want to add a little more chicken stock to moisten the couscous before serving if it seems a bit dry.

Chef's Secret

ABOUT TURMERIC
Turmeric comes in a powdered form and is actually a root, a member of the ginger family. It contains a bright yellow dye that gives its distinctive color to curries and other Asian dishes. It can also be used in place of saffron to give color to food but use it sparingly as it has a slightly bitter taste.

ORZO *with* PARMESAN CHEESE

Orzo is rice-shaped pasta that can be found at Italian or specialty shops. It's the perfect accompaniment to Tuscan Chicken (page 168) or any other Italian meat or fish dish.

2 cups (500 mL) raw orzo
¼ cup (60 mL) unsalted butter
4 to 6 Tbsp (60 to 90 mL) low-sodium chicken or vegetable stock
6 Tbsp (90 mL) grated Parmesan cheese
freshly ground pepper to taste
4 to 5 Tbsp (60 to 75 mL) finely chopped Italian parsley

1 OR 2 DAYS BEFORE Cook the orzo in a large Dutch oven with plenty of water for 10 to 12 minutes, or until barely tender and doubled in volume. Do not overcook. Drain well in a colander, rinsing with plenty of cold water to remove excess starch. Drain again. Melt the butter in a large, heavy frying pan. Add the orzo and heat through. Add just enough stock to moisten the orzo and then stir in the Parmesan cheese. Season with pepper to taste. Toss with the chopped parsley. Cover and refrigerate overnight.

TO SERVE Reheat covered with aluminum foil in a 350°F (180°C) oven for 35 to 40 minutes or until hot.

Serves 6

PER SERVING
130 calories
4 g protein
7 g fat
11 g carbohydrate
0 g fiber
57 mg sodium

Chef's Secret

KEEPING IT MOIST If you make this ahead, you might want to add a little more chicken stock and Parmesan cheese to moisten the orzo before reheating. Add sautéed mushrooms, prosciutto and roasted peppers and this dish makes a meal in itself.

PASTA *with* LEMON SAUCE, BASIL *and* MINT

....

PER SERVING
830 calories
30 g protein
40 g fat
97 g carbohydrate
9 g fiber
587 mg sodium

Chef's Secret

THE REAL THING I always use Italian Parmigiano Reggiano, and buy a chunk from the wheel and grate it fresh as I need it. You use less of this cheese as the quality is superior.

From Nancy and Chuck Kennedy's mountain Tuscan villa comes this sublime lemon pasta dish. So simple, so fresh. Serve as a side dish with Grilled Lemon Chicken with Red Pepper Chutney (page 171) or Marietta's Italian Roasted Chicken (page 172) and spring asparagus. *Magnifico!*

1 lb (500 g) dry linguine or tagliatelle pasta
½ cup (125 mL) olive oil
6 Tbsp (90 mL) lemon juice (about 3 lemons)
¼ cup (60 mL) chopped fresh basil
¼ cup (60 mL) finely chopped fresh mint
¼ cup (60 mL) finely chopped fresh Italian parsley
3 Tbsp (45 mL) lemon zest (about 3 lemons)
freshly ground pepper to taste
1 cup (250 mL) pasta stock
⅔ cup (150 mL) grated Parmesan cheese for garnish

Cook the pasta according to the package instructions. Meanwhile, mix the olive oil, lemon juice, basil, mint, parsley, lemon zest and pepper in a small bowl. Set aside. Drain the pasta, setting aside 1 cup (250 mL) of the pasta stock. In a large bowl, toss the pasta in the lemon mixture. Add some of the pasta stock if it seems a little dry. Serve immediately. Pass around a bowl of the grated Parmesan cheese at the table.

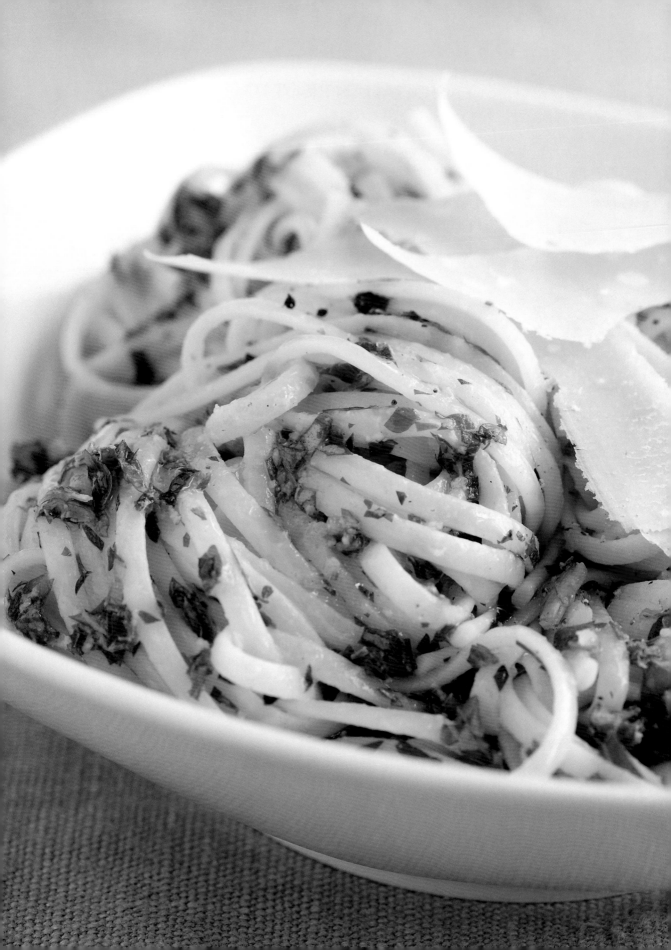

BASIC ITALIAN RISOTTO

Serves 6

....

PER SERVING
480 calories
20 g protein
22 g fat
54 g carbohydrate
4 g fiber
585 mg sodium

Risotto is one of my most popular dinner party entrées. In this recipe I've reduced the sodium content by using low-sodium chicken stock and reducing the amount of Parmesan cheese. The keys to a successful risotto are patience and the perfect rice to guarantee a creamy smooth texture. The best types of rice to use are carnaroli, vialone nano and arborio, because of their starchy qualities. I never tire of making risotto for an impromptu dinner party. You can get a head start on prepping the rice and then allow about 25 minutes to completion. It's worth every minute. Let your guests pitch in and give the risotto a stir while you're putting the final touches to the dinner. That's one way they'll learn the secrets to a successful risotto.

Chef's Secret

JAZZING UP BASIC RISOTTO To the basic Risotto recipe, during the last 15 minutes of cooking, add the last 2 cups (500 mL) of the chicken stock to the rice, then add 1 cup (250 mL) of the following choices to the risotto mixture: sautéed mushrooms, blanched asparagus pieces or fresh corn kernels, and sliced cooked chicken or raw prawns. Continue stirring until the rice and prawns are cooked and the rice is creamy. Add more stock if needed. Serve immediately.

2 to 3 Tbsp (30 to 45 mL) olive oil

½ cup (125 mL) finely chopped onions

½ cup (125 mL) finely chopped shallots

2 cloves of garlic, finely chopped

2½ cups (625 mL) raw arborio rice

1 cup (250 mL) dry white wine

7 to 8 cups (1.75 to 2 L) low-sodium chicken stock

⅓ cup (75 mL) grated Parmesan cheese

freshly ground pepper to taste

⅓ cup (75 mL) Italian mascarpone cheese or crème fraîche (optional)

SEVERAL HOURS BEFORE SERVING Warm the olive oil in a heavy saucepan over moderate heat and add the onions, shallots and garlic. Sauté for a few minutes until golden and translucent. Add the rice and stir for a few more minutes. You can prepare the rice to this stage earlier on the day of serving, or the night before (cover and refrigerate). Set aside until ready to commence the final preparation.

TO SERVE Add the white wine and stir until absorbed. Begin adding hot chicken stock, 1 ladle at a time, every few minutes, stirring all the while and keeping the rice at a constant simmer. Cook about 25 minutes, or until the rice is slightly *al dente* and the risotto is creamy. Add the Parmesan cheese during the last 5 minutes of cooking; add pepper to taste. Add more chicken stock if you think the risotto is too dry. Add the mascarpone cheese just before serving, if desired, for a creamier consistency. Offer extra Parmesan cheese in a bowl for your guests to sprinkle on top of the risotto.

TO REHEAT Leftover risotto can be reheated in a nonstick frying pan. For a tasty brunch, flip over to brown both sides, cut into wedges and serve topped with a poached egg.

BULGUR RICE PILAF

Chatelaine magazine featured this recipe in one of its issues and said, "It's the best bulgur wheat recipe we've tested!" The combination of cracked bulgur wheat and brown rice spiked with turmeric and lemon not only gives my dish a distinct flavor and nut-like texture, they make this winning pilaf a healthy and tasty choice. This recipe can be prepared a day ahead and reheated just before serving.

2 Tbsp (30 mL) unsalted butter

½ cup (125 mL) finely chopped onion

½ cup (125 mL) uncooked bulgur wheat

½ cup (125 mL) brown rice, washed and strained

½ tsp (2 mL) turmeric

2 cups (500 mL) low-sodium chicken stock, heated to boiling

⅓ cup (75 mL) raisins or dried currants (optional)

2 Tbsp (30 mL) chopped Italian parsley

1 Tbsp (15 mL) lemon juice

2 tsp (10 mL) lemon zest

⅓ cup (75 mL) finely chopped toasted pecans (optional)

freshly ground pepper to taste

1 OR 2 DAYS BEFORE Melt the butter in a large saucepan. Add the onion, bulgur, brown rice and turmeric, and sauté until golden, about 4 minutes. Add the chicken stock and raisins (if using). Cover and simmer for 30 to 35 minutes, until all the liquid is absorbed. Add the parsley, lemon juice and zest and pecans (if using); toss and serve. Or cool, cover and refrigerate.

TO SERVE Preheat the oven to 350°F (180°C) and reheat for 20 to 25 minutes, or until hot. Season with pepper and serve.

Serves 4 to 6

PER SERVING
235 calories
5 g protein
10 g fat
32 g carbohydrate
2 g fiber
52 mg sodium

Chef's Secret

BULGUR WHEAT Bulgur, used in North African and Lebanese cooking, is wheat berries that have been parboiled, dried and coarsely ground. Don't confuse bulgur with cracked wheat, which is simply that—cracked wheat.

SPEEDY REFRIED BEANS

Serves 8 to 12

PER SERVING
110 calories
6 g protein
4 g fat
13 g carbohydrate
3 g fiber
400 mg sodium

Serve these beans as a side dish with the Tex-Mex Salmon Tacos (page 177) or other Mexican dishes.

three 14 oz (398 mL) cans low-fat organic refried beans
½ cup (125 mL) Tomato and Red Onion Salsa (page 110)
2 tsp (10 mL) ground cumin
freshly ground pepper to taste
½ cup (125 mL) grated low-fat cheddar cheese
⅓ cup (75 mL) finely chopped green onions for garnish

Slightly mash the refried beans in a bowl. Add the Tomato and Red Onion Salsa, cumin and pepper. Put in a shallow 6-cup (1.5 L) casserole dish and top with the cheese. Cover and refrigerate until ready to reheat.

TO SERVE Preheat the oven to 350°F (180°C). Bake uncovered about 30 minutes or until hot and bubbly. The refried beans can also be heated in the microwave for 2 to 3 minutes. Just before serving, top with the chopped green onions.

CHINA GRILL VEGETABLE RICE

This is my version of a colourful dish from New York's famous restaurant, China Grill, which is the perfect complement to the Chicken Satay with Spicy Peanut Dip (page 136). Or try it alongside some of the dishes in the Asian Express menu (page 57).

(page 136). Or try it alongside some of the dishes in the Asian Express menu (page 57).

RICE

2½ cups (625 mL) brown rice

4 cups (1 L) water

VEGETABLES

1 cup (250 mL) finely diced carrots

1 cup (250 mL) thinly sliced (on the diagonal) asparagus

1 cup (250 mL) finely diced broccoli or broccolini

1 red pepper, finely diced

1 yellow pepper, finely diced

3 Tbsp (45 mL) vegetable oil

1 cup (250 mL) chopped green onion

½ cup (125 mL) chopped shallots

1 Tbsp (15 mL) finely chopped fresh ginger

3 cloves of garlic, finely chopped

¼ tsp (1 mL) red pepper flakes

1 large egg, slightly beaten (optional)

3 to 4 Tbsp (45 to 60 mL) low-sodium soy sauce

freshly ground pepper to taste

Serves 12

PER SERVING
220 calories
6 g protein
5 g fat
40 g carbohydrate
3 g fiber
240 mg sodium

Chef's Secret

VITAMIN AND CALCIUM GIANTS: EDAMAME AND BROCCOLINI If you want to add a boost of vitamins to this dish, add ½ cup (125 mL) of shelled and cooked edamame, or ½ cup (125 mL) or broccolini along with the other vegetables.

1 OR 2 DAYS BEFORE Prepare the rice. Rinse the uncooked rice and add the water. Bring to a boil and simmer about 40 minutes, or until all the liquid is absorbed. Check frequently after 20 minutes to make sure the rice is not sticking to the bottom. Cool, cover and refrigerate.

SEVERAL HOURS BEFORE SERVING Prepare the carrots, asparagus, broccoli and peppers. They must be very small cubes to cook quickly. Cover and refrigerate.

JUST BEFORE SERVING Warm a large wok or frying pan for 20 seconds over high heat and then add the oil. First add the diced carrots, sauté about 2 minutes and then add the asparagus, broccoli, red pepper, yellow pepper, green onion, shallots, ginger, garlic and red pepper flakes. Stir fry about 2 minutes. Add the beaten egg (if using) and stir. Add the cooked rice and continue to stir fry for 3 minutes. Shake the pan frequently. Add the soy sauce and pepper and continue to cook for another 30 to 45 seconds. Serve immediately. Leftovers can be reheated or frozen for later use.

VEGETARIAN CHILI

Serves 8 to 10

....

PER SERVING
375 calories
19 g protein
8 g fat
60 g carbohydrate
7 g fiber
680 mg sodium

When my daughter, Jennifer, and I opened the Tomato Fresh Food Café in 1991, the Vegetarian Chili became one of our most popular dishes. Served with my family's recipe for Champion Cornbread (page 158) it was a meal in itself. This chili contains absolutely everything that's good for you, including chunky vegetables full of vitamins, kidney beans and bulgur wheat for carbohydrates. It freezes well.

1½ cups (375 mL) dried red kidney beans

4 cups (1 L) cold water

¾ cup (190 mL) bulgur wheat

1½ cups (375 mL) boiling water

2 Tbsp (30 mL) vegetable oil

3 large cloves of garlic, finely chopped

1 large onion, chopped

1 cup (250 mL) ½-inch (1 cm) sliced celery

1 cup (250 mL) ½-inch (1 cm) sliced carrots

1 cup (250 mL) 1-inch (2.5 cm) cubed butternut squash (optional)

1 or 2 large green zucchini, halved lengthwise, cut into ½-inch (1 cm) slices

1 cup (250 mL) halved mushrooms

2 red peppers, cut into 1-inch (2.5 cm) squares

1 yellow pepper, cut into 1-inch (2.5 cm) squares

2 fresh jalapeño chilies, finely chopped

¼ cup (60 mL) fresh or 1 Tbsp (15 mL) dried basil

¼ cup (60 mL) fresh or 1 Tbsp (15 mL) dried dill

¼ cup (60 mL) fresh or 1 Tbsp (15 mL) dried oregano

3 Tbsp (45 mL) chili powder, or to taste

2 Tbsp (30 mL) ground cumin

½ tsp (2 mL) Tabasco sauce, or to taste

¼ tsp (1 mL) red pepper flakes, or to taste

one 28 oz (796 mL) can Italian plum tomatoes, chopped, with juice (about 3½ cups/875 mL)

3 cups (750 mL) vegetable juice

3 Tbsp (45 mL) tomato paste

1 cup (250 mL) corn niblets, fresh or frozen

½ cup (125 mL) grated low-fat cheddar cheese for garnish

½ cup (125 mL) grated low-fat Monterey Jack cheese for garnish

finely chopped red onions for garnish

1 OR 2 DAYS BEFORE Place the beans in a medium-sized pot and cover with the cold water. Bring to a boil and simmer 45 to 50 minutes, until tender. Strain, saving the liquid, and set aside. Soak the bulgur wheat in the boiling water about 5 minutes, until the liquid is absorbed. Set aside.

Warm the oil in a large stockpot over medium heat. Sauté the garlic, onion, celery, carrots and butternut squash (if using) until the vegetables are crisp-tender, about 15 minutes. Add the zucchini, mushrooms, peppers, chilies, basil, dill, oregano, chili powder, cumin, Tabasco and red pepper flakes. Sauté about 5 minutes. Add the tomatoes with juice, vegetable juice and tomato paste, and then add the reserved beans and bean liquid. Simmer over medium heat about 30 minutes, uncovered, until the vegetables are still slightly crunchy. Add the corn and reserved bulgur wheat. Check for seasonings. Cool and chill overnight until ready to serve.

TO SERVE Reheat over medium heat uncovered, stirring frequently until hot. Serve in bowls, topped with the grated cheeses and chopped red onions.

Chef's Secret

MAKE IT WITH MEAT If you'd like a nonvegetarian version, add 1 lb (500 g) of browned ground turkey or chicken just before adding the tomatoes.

CHAMPION CORNBREAD

Makes 8 generous pieces

PER SERVING
304 calories
13 g protein
9 g fat
42 g carbohydrate
1 g fiber
699 mg sodium

Chef's Secret

CORNBREAD IN THE TEST KITCHEN "Dynamite cornbread," is the comment I love to hear every time I whip up a batch of this cornbread. After our family and friends had devoured 200 pans and 1,600 or more pieces, I finally had a winning recipe.

This is a hearty cornbread made with cornmeal, corn niblets, cheddar and a hint of green chilies. It's the ideal match for Vegetarian Chili (page 156), or for soups or summer barbecues. Quick to make, it's best served hot from the oven, or made a day ahead and reheated, as it doesn't freeze well. Don't be surprised by the amount of baking powder.

2½ cups (625 mL) all-purpose flour
1½ cups (375 mL) 100% stone-ground wholegrain yellow cornmeal
3 Tbsp (45 mL) baking powder
2 cups (500 mL) low-fat buttermilk
1 cup (250 mL) corn niblets, thawed or frozen
1 cup (250 mL) grated low-fat cheddar cheese
one 4 oz (113 g) can chopped mild green chilies
3 large eggs, slightly beaten
¼ cup (60 mL) melted unsalted butter

THE DAY BEFORE Preheat the oven to 350°F (180°C) and lightly grease a 13- by 9-inch (3.5 L) baking pan with vegetable oil. In a large mixing bowl, whisk together the flour, cornmeal and baking powder. Add the buttermilk, corn, cheese, chilies, eggs and butter, and mix just until blended. Do not overbeat. Spoon the thick batter into the pan. Bake about 40 to 50 minutes, or until a skewer inserted in the center of the loaf comes out clean and the top is golden brown. Check the middle to make sure it's cooked. Remove from the oven and serve, or cover and refrigerate overnight. Reheat just before serving.

TO REHEAT Wrap the loaf in aluminum foil and place in a 350°F (180°C) oven about 15 to 20 minutes, or until heated through. Try grilling the bread on the barbecue.

PITA CRISPS

Great for dips, spreads and salads, these crisps stay fresh for 1 to 2 weeks and boast only 30 calories per piece, making them great for munching. Prepare them plain, or spice them up with the tasty Pepper Sumac and Cumin Rub, which everyone loves.

PEPPER, SUMAC AND CUMIN RUB (OPTIONAL)

¼ cup (60 mL) freshly ground pepper

1 Tbsp (15 mL) plus 1 tsp (5 mL) ground sumac

½ tsp (2 mL) ground cumin

CRISPS

six 6-inch (15 cm) whole wheat pita wraps

olive oil for brushing

Prepare the Pepper, Sumac and Cumin Rub. Combine the pepper, ground sumac and ground cumin. Any leftover spice can be stored in a sealed jar for up to 6 months.

Prepare the Pita Crisps. Preheat the oven to 350°F (180°C). Cut the pita wraps in half horizontally. Brush the tops with a little of the olive oil. Sprinkle the tops with a little of the Pepper, Sumac and Cumin Rub (if using). Cut each half into 5 or 6 triangles. Bake on baking sheets in a single layer (you'll need 2 baking sheets) about 15 minutes, or until golden and crisp. Cool and store in an airtight container for up to 1 week.

Makes about 60

PER SERVING (6 CRISPS)
186 calories
5 g protein
10 g fat
21 g carbohydrate
1 g fiber
282 mg sodium

Chef's Secret

SPREADING THE RUB The Pepper, Sumac and Cumin Rub is also excellent sprinkled on Grilled Lemon Chicken with Red Pepper Chutney (page 171), Jane's Grilled Tuna Salad with Mango Pineapple Salsa (page 93) or other seafood and meats.

CROUTONS

Makes 6 cups (1.5 L)

PER SERVING
210 calories
0 g protein
23 g fat
2 g carbohydrate
0 g fiber
24 mg sodium

Chef's Secret

ARE THEY CRISPY? You can test whether croutons are cooked through and crispy by dropping 1 into a cup of water. If it floats it's done, but if it sinks to the bottom then it needs more time in the oven.

Normally croutons are brushed with calorie-laden olive oil and then baked. Over the years I've gone from using ½ cup (125 mL) olive oil to make croutons to now limiting the total amount to 2 to 3 Tbsp (30 to 45 mL)— a monumental difference in the nutritional analysis. I also use whole wheat bread. To our delight, the croutons are crunchy, light and good for you. Make a batch of whole wheat croutons to add to all your tossed salads and Gazpacho (page 81). They're also perfect for Caesar salad made with Low-Fat Caesar Dressing (page 105).

6 cups (1 to 1.5 L) small cubes of day-old whole wheat bread

2 to 3 Tbsp (30 to 45 mL) olive oil

freshly ground pepper to taste

Toss the whole wheat bread cubes in a large bowl with just enough olive oil to coat. Sprinkle with ground pepper to taste. Arrange on a baking sheet. Bake at 250°F (120°C) about 25 to 30 minutes or until golden. Toss frequently. Cool and refrigerate in a sealed container for 2 or 3 weeks.

CROSTINI

Crostini are simply thin slices of day-old Italian or French bread that have been baked in the oven or on a grill to serve as a base for tasty toppings. *Fetuntas* are crostini that have been rubbed with a little olive oil and garlic before grilling or baking. I prefer to make crostini rather than *fetuntas*.

1 average baguette makes about 24 crostini

1 sourdough or French whole wheat baguette

1 OR 2 DAYS BEFORE Preheat the oven to 350°F (180°C). Cut the baguette into ⅓-inch (8 mm) slices, on the diagonal or straight across. Place on a baking sheet and bake about 3 minutes on each side, or until crisp. Cool and store in airtight containers for up to 3 to 4 days.

protein catch-up

Meats, Poultry and Fish

MEDITERRANEAN RACK OF LAMB

As you've probably gathered, Doug and I enjoy lamb. Try the Mediterranean Rub (page 113) on your next rack of lamb as a change from the traditional breadcrumb coating. Serve with Potatoes Gratin (page 146) and Roasted Tomatoes (page 145) and Roasted Asparagus (page 144) to round out the main entrée.

2 racks of lamb, French-cut (trimmed of fat), allowing 2 to 3 small loins per person

1 large egg, slightly beaten

Mediterranean Rub (page 113)

A FEW HOURS BEFORE Dip the lamb racks in the beaten egg. Pat the Mediterranean Rub evenly over the 2 racks of lamb. Cover and refrigerate. Take the racks of lamb out of the refrigerator about 30 minutes before roasting.

TO SERVE Put the lamb racks in a roasting pan. Preheat the oven to 400°F (200°C). Roast about 30 minutes for medium doneness. Slice each rack and serve.

Serves 4

PER SERVING
317 calories
18 g protein
23 g fat
9 g carbohydrate
2 g fiber
90 mg sodium

Chef's Secret

FRENCH-CUT RACK OF LAMB Order your racks of lamb a few days before serving, and make sure the butcher "French cuts" them to eliminate the fat. Try the Mediterranean Rub on fillet of beef or pork tenderloin as well.

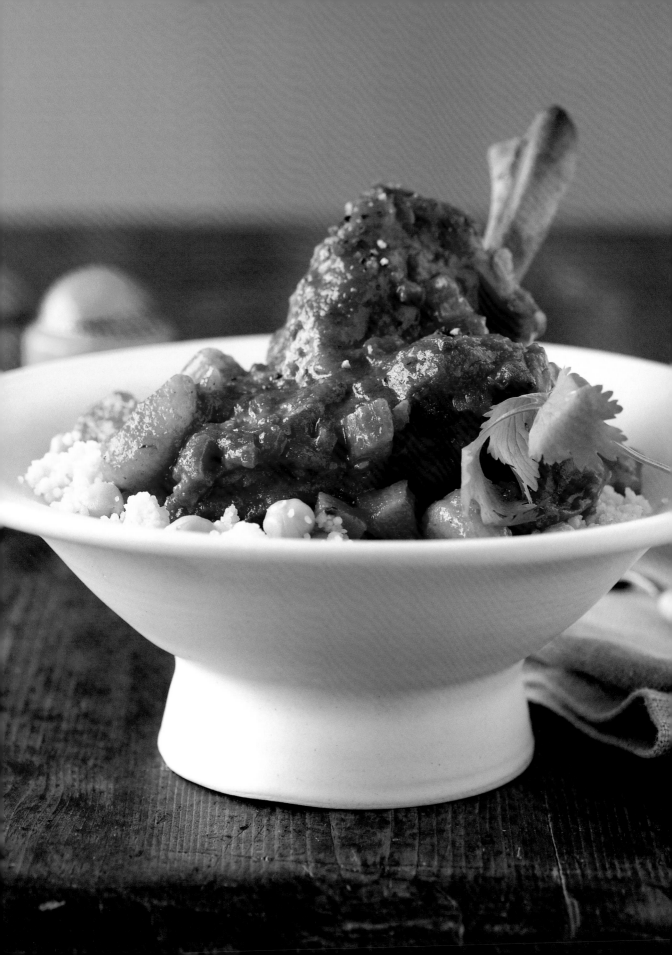

LAMB TAGINE *with* GLAZED CINNAMON FIGS

This is my choice for a luscious do-ahead Moroccan dinner (see menu on page 56). The lamb shanks just fall off the bone, and the Moroccan spice mix Ras-El-Hanout (page 112) will tantalize your taste buds. Serve with Couscous with Chickpeas (page 148).

LAMB TAGINE

¼ cup (60 mL) olive oil

6 lamb shanks, each 1 lb (500 g), fat trimmed

1½ cups (375 mL) finely chopped onions

½ cup (125 mL) finely chopped carrots

¼ cup (60 mL) finely chopped celery

4 cloves of garlic, finely chopped

⅓ cup (75 mL) lemon juice

1 recipe of Ras-El-Hanout (page 112)

freshly ground pepper to taste

one 28 oz (796 mL) can whole peeled tomatoes, drained and coarsely chopped

3 cups (750 mL) low-fat chicken stock

1 cup (250 mL) dry red wine

¼ cup (60 mL) tomato paste

1 cup (250 mL) apricots, cut in half

1 cup (250 mL) pitted dates, cut in half

¼ cup (60 mL) finely chopped Italian parsley

GLAZED CINNAMON FIGS

1 lb (500 g) dried figs

2 Tbsp (30 mL) olive oil

1 Tbsp (15 mL) cinnamon

1 Tbsp (15 mL) icing sugar

CONTINUED ON NEXT PAGE

Serves 6 to 8

PER SERVING
501 calories
19 g protein
22 g fat
56 g carbohydrate
7 g fiber
320 mg sodium

Chef's Secret

TAGINES The word *tagine* refers to both the contents and the container for this meat stew. A tagine dish is made from glazed clay and has a lid like a pointed hat that allows the steam to circulate inside. A Dutch oven works well in place of the traditional tagine dish. This dish freezes for up to 3 months. Take out of the freezer a day before serving and thaw in the refrigerator.

1 OR 2 DAYS BEFORE Prepare the Lamb Tagine. Preheat the oven to 350°F (180°C). Warm 2 Tbsp (30 mL) of the olive oil in a large Dutch oven over medium-high heat. Sauté the lamb in batches until browned all over. Add 1 Tbsp (15 mL) more olive oil if needed. Remove the lamb and set aside. Clean out the pan. Add the remaining 1 Tbsp (15 mL) olive oil to the pan. Add the onions, carrots, celery and garlic. Sauté for 3 to 4 minutes until slightly softened. Add the lemon juice, spice mixture and pepper to the pan. Sauté for 2 to 3 more minutes so that the spices blend with the vegetables. Add the tomatoes, chicken stock, red wine and tomato paste. Cover the Dutch oven and bake about 2 to 2½ hours, stirring occasionally. Add the apricots and dates. Cover and bake another ½ hour, stir and then continue to cook another ½ hour or so, or until the lamb is tender and falling off the bone. Cool, cover and refrigerate.

THE DAY BEFORE Prepare the Glazed Cinnamon Figs. Place the figs in a saucepan and cover them with boiling water. Cover and boil about 15 minutes. Drain and slice in half from top to bottom. Warm the oil, cinnamon and icing sugar in a frying pan over low heat. Add the figs and caramelize about 8 to 10 minutes on low heat, turning frequently to glaze. Serve at room temperature.

TO SERVE Cover the tagine and reheat at 350°F (180°C) for 30 minutes. Uncover and bake another 15 minutes, or until hot. If you're serving this with the Couscous with Chickpeas (page 148), heat it up at the same time. Garnish with fresh parsley and serve with the Glazed Cinnamon Figs.

PORK TENDERLOIN SUPERB

I rely on pork tenderloin for a quick-to-prepare meat accompaniment when entertaining. Make preparation even faster by picking up the tapenade at your deli. Serve with Potatoes Gratin (page 146), or Green Beans with Shiitake Mushrooms (page 141).

3 pork tenderloins, each 1 lb (500 g)	
1½ cups (375 mL) olive tapenade	
2 Tbsp (30 mL) Spanish sweet paprika	
freshly ground pepper to taste	
6 oz (175 g) thinly sliced pancetta	
2 Tbsp (30 mL) olive oil	
Roasted Red Pepper Sauce (page 107)	

EARLY ON THE DAY OF SERVING Trim and clean the tenderloins. Pat dry. Slice down the side of each loin but not all the way through. Lay on sheets of plastic wrap and cover with plastic wrap. Flatten with a meat mallet or the back of a wide knife to butterfly the loins. Spread ¼ cup (60 mL) of the tapenade down the length of each loin and fold over. Sprinkle the loins with paprika and pepper. Wrap the pancetta slices evenly around each loin, pressing tightly. Tie with kitchen string to hold them together. Warm the oil in a frying pan over medium-high heat. Sear the loins all over until browned. Cover and refrigerate until ready to roast and serve.

TO SERVE Take the loins out of the refrigerator 30 minutes before roasting. Preheat the oven to 375°F (190°C). Put in a roasting pan and roast about 35 to 40 minutes, or until no pink juices remain and a meat thermometer reads 160°F (71°C). Remove the string and slice thinly on the diagonal. Serve with the Roasted Red Pepper Sauce.

Serves 8

PER SERVING
679 calories
54 g protein
49 g fat
6 g carbohydrate
1 g fiber
434 mg sodium

Chef's Secret
FILLET OF BEEF SUPERB
Substitute fillet of beef for the pork tenderloin. Cut the amount of beef to 2 lbs (1 kg) and increase the oven temperature to 400°F (200°C). Roast about 30 to 35 minutes for medium rare or 125°F (52°C) on a meat thermometer.

TUSCAN CHICKEN

Serves 8

....

PER SERVING

540 calories

60 g protein

15 g fat

23 g carbohydrate

7 g fiber

155 mg sodium

I rely on this dish from central Italy for informal entertaining when I'm on the run! Both the chicken and the Orzo with Parmesan Cheese (page 149), which I like to serve with this dish, can be prepared ahead of time. I pick up several antipasto items from my favorite deli, along with rustic breads, biscotti and 2 or 3 sorbets. Pick up a few robust Italian wines as well and with very little effort we are ready to entertain.

⅓ cup (75 mL) olive oil

8 chicken breasts, boned, skinned and cut in half

2 onions, finely chopped

1½ cups (375 mL) dry white wine

1 cup (250 mL) sun-dried tomatoes in oil, drained and then cut into thin julienne strips

⅓ cup (75 mL) balsamic vinegar

freshly ground pepper to taste

1 cup (250 mL) thin julienne strips of basil, plus more for garnish

1 OR 2 DAYS AHEAD Warm 3 Tbsp (45 mL) of the olive oil in a large frying pan over medium heat. Sauté the chicken breasts, a few at a time, about 3 minutes on each side until just opaque, with no pink juices. Place in a shallow 13- by 9-inch (3.5 L) casserole dish. Cover and refrigerate while you prepare the onions. Add the remaining 2 Tbsp (30 mL) olive oil to the chicken pan. Toss in the onions and sauté 5 to 8 minutes, until slightly caramelized and deep golden. Add the wine, sun-dried tomatoes, balsamic vinegar and pepper. Simmer about 10 minutes to reduce the sauce and thicken slightly. Add the basil and pour evenly over the chicken. Cover and refrigerate.

TO SERVE Preheat the oven to 350°F (180°C) and bake about 30 minutes, or until the chicken is heated through. Sprinkle more basil on top, and serve with Orzo with Parmesan Cheese (page 149) or other pastas.

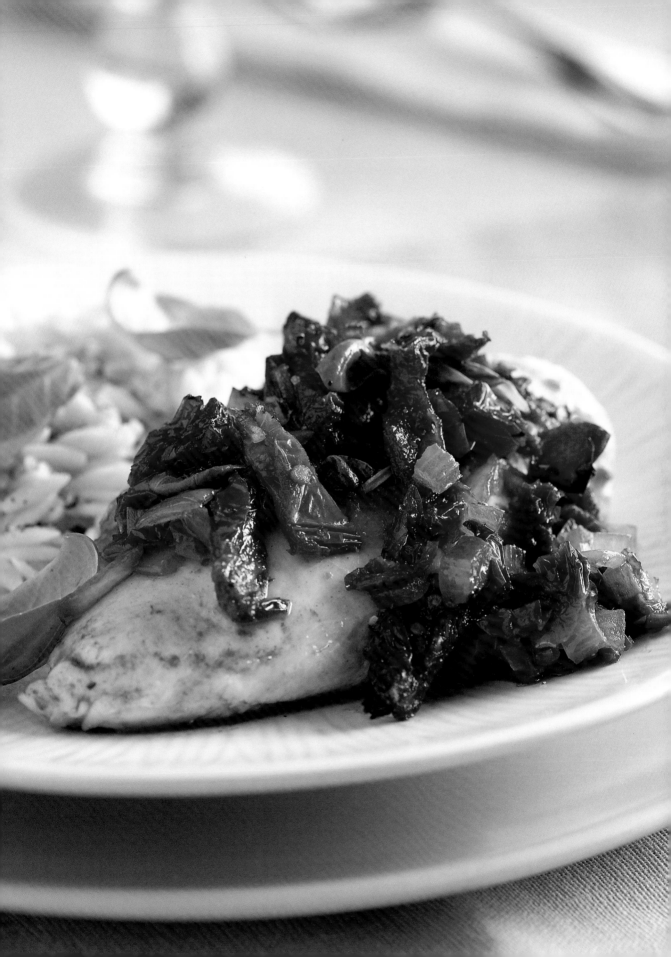

CHICKEN SALTIMBOCCA

Serves 6

PER SERVING
475 calories
57 g protein
23 g fat
11 g carbohydrate
2 g fiber
410 mg sodium

Chef's Secret

ORGANIC OR FREE-RANGE?
The key to a moist chicken
is to buy a good-quality
bird. An organic or free-
range chicken may cost
more, but it will have been
reared to high standards.

I love to serve this Italian classic recipe with the Pasta with Lemon Sauce, Basil and Mint (page 150), Orzo with Parmesan Cheese (page 149) or Basic Italian Risotto (page 152).

BREADCRUMB COATING

⅓ cup (75 mL) fine dry Italian breadcrumbs

3 Tbsp (45 mL) grated Parmesan cheese

3 Tbsp (45 mL) finely chopped Italian parsley

2 Tbsp (30 mL) olive oil

½ tsp (2 mL) herbes de Provence (page 140)

6 boneless, skinned chicken breasts

6 thin slices prosciutto

5 oz (150 g) mozzarella or fontina cheese, cut into 6 thin slices

6 Roma tomatoes, peeled, seeded and thinly sliced

12 basil leaves

A FEW HOURS BEFORE Prepare the coating by combining the breadcrumbs, cheese, parsley, olive oil and herbs in a bowl. Set aside.

Prepare the chicken breasts. Cover the chicken with plastic wrap and pound with a meat mallet or the flat side of a large carving knife to an even thickness. Place a slice each of the ham and cheese to fit on each breast. Top with 2 or 3 tomato slices and a layer of 2 basil leaves. Press down, tuck in the sides and roll up jelly-roll fashion, pressing to seal. Secure with toothpicks. Roll each piece in the Breadcrumb Coating. Place in a shallow baking pan. Cover and refrigerate until ready to bake.

TO SERVE Preheat the oven to 350°F (180°C). Bake about 25 to 30 minutes. Remove the toothpicks. Slice the chicken in half on the diagonal to serve.

GRILLED LEMON CHICKEN
with RED PEPPER CHUTNEY

I was invited to special luncheon at the Four Seasons Hotel in Vancouver, prepared by the executive chef and a guest from California's Mondovi Winery. This recipe is my adaptation of the light chicken dish that was served. I like to serve it with Pasta with Lemon Sauce, Basil and Mint (page 150) or Potatoes Gratin (page 146). The Red Pepper Chutney also goes well with grilled seafood.

CHICKEN MARINADE

juice of 4 lemons

2 Tbsp (30 mL) Dijon mustard

1 Tbsp (15 mL) lemon zest

freshly ground pepper to taste

6 single chicken breasts, boned and skinned

RED PEPPER CHUTNEY

6 Tbsp (90 mL) raspberry vinegar

¼ cup (60 mL) white sugar

4 large tomatoes, peeled, seeded and chopped

3 red peppers, grilled, peeled and chopped

AT LEAST 2 TO 4 HOURS BEFORE Prepare the chicken. Whisk together the lemon juice, mustard, lemon zest and pepper in a small bowl just until blended. Place the chicken breasts in a single layer in a 13- by 9-inch (3.5 L) casserole dish. Pour the marinade over the chicken breasts. Cover and refrigerate for 2 to 4 hours.

Prepare the Red Pepper Chutney. Mix the vinegar and sugar in a small frying pan over low to medium heat. Simmer until the mixture begins to form a thin syrup and the sugar begins to caramelize. Add the tomatoes and red peppers. Stir to blend, and simmer on low heat until slightly thickened. Set aside at room temperature.

TO SERVE Grill the chicken breasts on the barbecue or under the broiler about 6 to 8 minutes on each side, or until cooked and no pink juices show. Reheat the Red Pepper Chutney slightly and serve with the chicken.

Serves 6

PER SERVING
240 calories
34 g protein
2 g fat
20 g carbohydrate
3 g fiber
280 mg sodium

Chef's Secret

BE PREPARED Prepare 3 or 4 extra chicken breasts to tuck in the freezer for quick stir fries, pasta or sandwiches.

MARIETTA'S ITALIAN ROASTED CHICKEN

Serves 8

PER SERVING
500 calories
50 g protein
24 g fat
12 g carbohydrate
2 g fiber
440 mg sodium

When Doug and I were hosting with Italian restaurateur Umberto Menghi at his famous Villa Delia Cooking School in Tuscany, Umberto's sister, Marietta, teased our palates with this succulent chicken dish. Her enthusiastic husband, Silvano, served it to us with pride! This is my version of her winning dish. Always a favorite for Sunday dinner, with extra for sandwiches the next day, or freeze for stir fries or casseroles.

2 whole roasting chickens, about 2 lb (1 kg) each

freshly ground pepper to taste

4 lemons, cut in half (2 lemons per bird)

10 cloves of garlic, peeled (5 per bird)

2 to 4 small sage branches (1 large or 2 small per bird) plus more to surround the birds

olive oil for rubbing

1 cup (250 mL) low-sodium chicken stock

lemon zest and sage leaves for garnish (optional)

Chef's Secret

CHICKEN SIZZLER Marietta roasts her chicken at a higher temperature and for less time than usual. It works for me, too! The high temperature and the water added to the pan produce a moist chicken. The lemons keep the chicken succulent and the citrus sage sauce is truly a taste of Italy.

Preheat the oven to 450°F (230°C). Remove the giblets and neck from the chickens. Rinse well and pat dry. Sprinkle the birds inside and out with pepper. Place the lemon halves, garlic and sage leaves in the cavities. Rub olive oil over the birds. Place on a rack in a large roasting pan. Add more sage leaves around the birds. Add water to the pan to about the 1-inch (2.5 cm) level. Roast until the interior temperature of the chickens reaches 160°F to 165°F (71°C to 74°C) on a meat thermometer, or until the legs are soft and there are no pink juices, about 1½ hours. Add more water to the pan as needed. Remove the chickens from the pan, reserving the juices. Squeeze the juice from the lemons into the pan and mash the garlic and add it to the pan. Add the chicken stock and bring to a boil. Strain.

TO SERVE Cut the chicken into pieces and pour the juices overtop. Sprinkle each plate with a little lemon zest and sage leaves, if desired.

CHICKEN TORTILLA PIE

A do-ahead Mexican casserole to take to the ski slopes or to serve for any casual weekend of entertaining. Include the condiment ideas from the Tex-Mex Salmon Taco Party menu (page 55). Easy to whip up, this is one of our family's all-time favorites. To revise this casserole to meet our health-friendly mandate, I've chosen low-fat and low-sodium chicken stock and lower-in-fat cheese. This change has reduced the overall caloric intake, but the good news is that you'd never know the difference from the original taste of the pie.

2 Tbsp (30 mL) vegetable oil

½ cup (125 mL) finely chopped onions

2 cloves of garlic, finely chopped

two 4 oz (113 g) cans chopped mild green chilies (about 1 cup/250 mL)

1 cup (250 mL) enchilada sauce or medium taco sauce

1 cup (250 mL) canned tomato or marinara sauce

1 cup (250 mL) low-fat chicken stock

1 cup (250 mL) skim milk

1½ cups (375 mL) grated low-fat Monterey Jack cheese

¼ tsp (1 mL) dried red chili peppers

freshly ground pepper to taste

3 cups (750 mL) cooked chicken breast or 1 whole cooked chicken, cut in strips

eighteen 6-inch (15 cm) corn tortillas

1 cup (250 mL) grated low-fat old cheddar cheese

Serves 8 to 10

PER SERVING
327 calories
28 g protein
11 g fat
28 g carbohydrate
2 g fiber
575 mg sodium

Chef's Secret
Save time and pick up the cooked chicken from your favorite deli.

THE DAY BEFORE Warm the oil in a frying pan over medium heat. Sauté the onions and garlic a few minutes until softened. Add the chilies, sauces, stock, milk, chili peppers and Monterey Jack cheese. Stir until the cheese is melted. Add pepper to taste, and then the chicken. (It may look a little curdled, but the cheese will melt when baked.) Preheat the oven to 350°F (180°C). Lightly grease a 13- by 9-inch (3.5 L) casserole dish with vegetable oil. Place 6 tortillas in the bottom, overlapping a little. Cover with a third of the chicken mixture, then another layer of tortillas. Repeat the layers, ending with a layer of the chicken mixture on top. Sprinkle with the cheddar cheese. Bake about 30 to 40 minutes. Cool, cover and refrigerate.

TO SERVE Reheat at 350°F (180°C), covered with aluminum foil, about 30 to 40 minutes or until heated through. Remove the foil during the last few minutes of cooking.

TEQUILA CHICKEN

Serves 6

PER SERVING
397 calories
54 g protein
6 g fat
5 g carbohydrate
1 g fiber
141 mg sodium

Try this fun Mexican marinade for chicken tacos that we enjoyed during our stay in Cabo San Lucas. Serve it with other dishes on the Tex-Mex Salmon Taco Party menu (page 55) in place of the salmon.

TEQUILA MARINADE

1 cup (250 mL) tequila

½ cup (125 mL) orange juice

3 Tbsp (45 mL) lime juice

1 Tbsp (15 mL) chili powder

4 cloves of garlic, coarsely chopped

2 jalapeño peppers, seeded and finely chopped

freshly ground pepper to taste

6 boneless and skinless chicken breasts

12 corn tacos, allowing 2 tacos per person

THE DAY BEFORE Prepare the Tequila Marinade. Combine the tequila, orange juice, lime juice, chili powder, garlic, jalapeños and pepper in a large bowl. Add the chicken breasts. Cover and marinate in the refrigerator overnight.

TO SERVE To barbecue, set the barbecue to medium heat. Place the chicken on the grill and sear for 5 minutes per side, or until there are no pink juices and the temperature reads 170°F (77°C) on a meat thermometer. Alternatively, cook the chicken in a grill pan on the stovetop over medium-high heat. Slice into thin strips and serve with corn tacos.

HALIBUT TUSCAN STYLE

When fresh halibut is available, enjoy this quick-to-prepare Tuscan dish.
Or substitute sablefish, red snapper or cod with equal success. Vegetable
Gratin (page 139) makes a colorful side dish, so prepare it early on the day
of serving and refrigerate. Pop it in the oven while you prep the fish. Local
new baby potatoes, green beans or asparagus are other tasty vegetable choices.

2 Tbsp (30 mL) olive oil

½ cup (125 mL) sliced onion

3 cloves of garlic, finely chopped

four 5 oz (150 g) fillets of halibut, skinned and boned

one 19 oz (540 mL) can diced tomatoes

½ cup (125 mL) pitted, halved black olives

½ cup (125 mL) dry white wine

¼ cup (60 mL) chopped Italian parsley

¼ cup (60 mL) chopped basil

pinch of red pepper flakes

freshly ground pepper to taste

Serves 4

PER SERVING
322 calories
32 g protein
15 g fat
11 g carbohydrate
0 g fiber
690 mg sodium

Warm the oil in a frying pan over medium heat. Add the onion and garlic,
and sauté until softened, about 2 minutes. Add the fish. Cook about 2 minutes
or until slightly golden. Turn the fish and cook an additional 2 minutes. Add
the tomatoes, olives, wine, parsley, basil, red pepper flakes and pepper, and
simmer covered for another 8 to 10 minutes, basting the fish from time to
time. When the fish is opaque, remove to 4 plates. Spoon the sauce from the
pan over the fish.

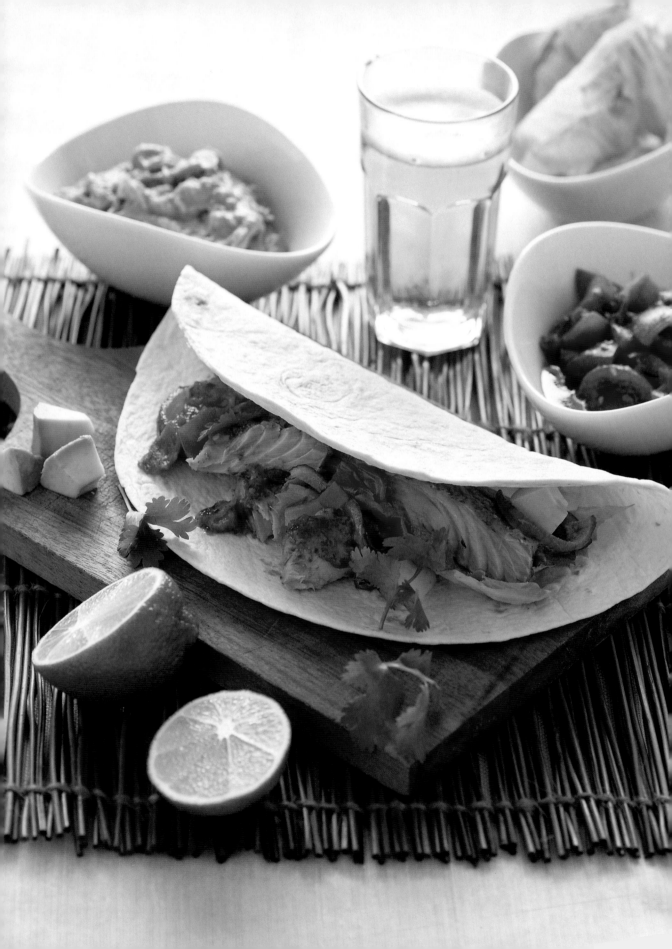

TEX-MEX SALMON TACOS

For the family on the run, what could be easier for weekend entertaining with friends or family than a Mexican taco party? Most of this Tex-Mex Salmon Taco Party menu (page 55) is done ahead of time, with guests and family creating their own tacos. It's an easy, fun party for the hosts to enjoy. Salmon, marinated in the tangy Tex-Mex Seasoning, is the star attraction, a healthy and tasty choice.

TEX-MEX SEASONING

3 Tbsp (45 mL) ground cumin

3 Tbsp (45 mL) ground coriander

1 Tbsp (15 mL) chili powder

freshly ground pepper to taste

MARINADE FOR SALMON

¼ cup (60 mL) Tex-Mex Seasoning

¼ cup (60 mL) honey

2 Tbsp (30 mL) grainy mustard

1 Tbsp (15 mL) red wine vinegar

SALMON TACOS

2 lb (1 kg) skinned wild salmon fillets (eight 1-inch/2.5 cm thick fillets, about 4 oz/125 g each)

sixteen 8-inch (20 cm) flour tortillas, folded into quarters

GARNISH

3 cups (750 mL) thinly sliced iceberg lettuce

5 limes, sliced into wedges

1 bunch cilantro

CONTINUED ON NEXT PAGE

Serves 8 to 12

PER SERVING
290 calories
23 g protein
10 g fat
28 g carbohydrate
3 g fiber
115 mg sodium

1 OR 2 DAYS BEFORE Prepare the Tex-Mex Seasoning. Combine the cumin, coriander, chili powder and pepper in a small bowl. Store in a sealed container. Will keep for 3 months in a cool place.

EARLY ON THE DAY OF SERVING Prepare the Marinade for Salmon. Blend the Tex-Mex Seasoning, honey, mustard and vinegar, in a small bowl. Set aside.

Place the salmon fillets in a shallow baking dish. Pour the marinade evenly over the salmon fillets. Turn the fillets over to coat well. Cover and refrigerate.

JUST BEFORE SERVING Preheat the oven to 350°F (180°C). Wrap the tortillas in aluminum foil and heat about 10 minutes until warm. Remove and set aside to keep warm while grilling the salmon on medium-high heat for 5 to 7 minutes.

Preheat the broiler. Place the salmon on a baking sheet. Broil without turning until opaque, about 5 minutes. Cool. If you prefer, barbecue the fillets of salmon.

TO SERVE Arrange the cooked salmon fillets, lettuce, limes and cilantro on a large platter. Serve with the warmed tortillas and Guacamole (page 135), salsas and corn chips. Let everyone dig in and create their own tacos. Start with breaking the salmon fillet in bite-sized pieces and adding the condiments. Serve with Speedy Refried Beans (page 154) on the side.

CAMPBELL RIVER GRILLED SALMON

Dr. Bob and Jacquie Gordon invited us to an unbelievable salmon barbecue on Vancouver Island on the final promotion tour for my first cookbook, *Chef on the Run*. This recipe was given to Bob and Jacquie by their friend, a former First Nations Chief in Campbell River, who revealed his secret recipe for the most succulent salmon I've ever eaten. The combination of soy sauce, brown sugar and a hint of whiskey gives the salmon its slightly smoked flavor. Try halibut, Alaska cod (sable fish) or red snapper as well.

one 2 lb (1 kg) salmon fillet with skin on, or six 5 oz (150 g) salmon fillets steaks

MARINADE

½ cup (125 mL) vegetable oil

¼ cup (60 mL) whiskey

2 Tbsp (30 mL) brown sugar

2 Tbsp (30 mL) low-sodium soy sauce

3 cloves of garlic, finely chopped

freshly ground pepper to taste

lemon wedges for garnish

SEVERAL HOURS BEFORE Wipe the fish and set aside. Combine the vegetable oil, whiskey, sugar, soy sauce, garlic and pepper to make a marinade. Pour the marinade over the fish, reserving some for basting, and leave it to steep about 2 hours.

TO SERVE Set the barbecue grill to medium, oil the grill and barbecue the salmon. Or broil on high in your oven for about 4 minutes per side, just until the fish flakes. Brush with the remaining marinade several times during cooking. Serve with wedges of lemon.

Serves 6

PER SERVING
410 calories
26 g protein
25 g fat
4 g carbohydrate
0 g fiber
270 mg sodium

Chef's Secret

QUICK FISH FOR DINNER
Preheat the oven broiler to high. Drizzle a 4 to 5 oz (125 to 150 g) fillet of salmon, halibut or cod with a little olive oil, and sprinkle with freshly ground pepper to taste and a squeeze of lemon juice. Put on a baking pan and broil 4 to 5 inches (10 to 12 cm) from the heat, turning once, for 10 to 12 minutes, until the flesh is flaky and opaque. Or preheat the oven to 400°F (200°C) and bake about 15 to 20 minutes, turning once.

treat time

Desserts

LIME MOUSSE *with* TROPICAL FRUIT

Almost a piña colada, this refreshing dessert version of the popular drink is dynamite. A favorite after-dinner treat from our first *Chef and Doctor on the Run* cookbook, published in 1986, it still boasts only 100 calories per serving.

LIME MOUSSE

¼ cup (60 mL) unsweetened pineapple juice

1 Tbsp (15 mL) unflavored gelatin (1 packet)

¾ cup (175 mL) frozen limeade concentrate, thawed but not diluted

2 Tbsp (30 mL) canned light cream of coconut milk

1 Tbsp (15 mL) white rum (optional)

1 cup (250 mL) low-fat plain yogurt

3 large egg whites

pinch of cream of tartar

TROPICAL FRUIT

1 mango, peeled, seeded and coarsely chopped

1 pineapple, peeled, cored and coarsely chopped

2 kiwis, peeled and coarsely chopped

THE DAY BEFORE Prepare the Lime Mousse. Combine the pineapple juice and gelatin in a small saucepan. Stir until smooth. Let the mixture sit until it starts to firm. Turn the heat to low and stir well until the gelatin melts. Add the limeade, coconut milk and rum (if using) and mix well. Pour into a glass bowl. Chill until the mousse thickens, about 30 minutes. Check often so that it doesn't get too stiff. Fold in the yogurt and combine well. Whip the egg whites until foamy and add the cream of tartar. Whip until very stiff. Fold a little of the gelatin mixture into the egg whites and then fold in the rest. Do not overmix; there should still be a few streaks of white remaining. Spoon into 8 martini glasses or parfait dishes. Refrigerate until ready to serve.

Prepare the Tropical Fruit. Mix the mango, pineapple and kiwis in a small bowl. Cover and refrigerate.

TO SERVE Top each dessert with a little Tropical Fruit.

Serves 8

PER SERVING
100 calories
4 g protein
2 g fat
16 g carbohydrate
2 g fiber
45 mg sodium

Chef's Secret

LEFTOVER COCONUT MILK Freeze leftover coconut milk in ice cube trays and then put in sealed plastic bags. Take out when needed to add to stir fried Asian vegetables, fruit smoothies or dessert mousses.

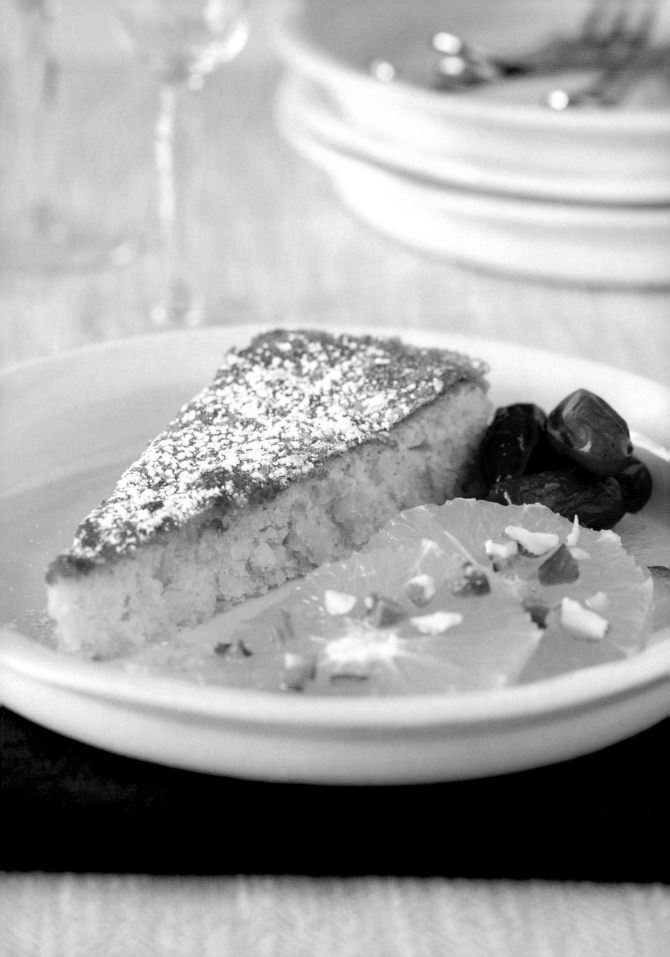

SPANISH ALMOND TART *with* ORANGE *and* DATE COMPOTE

In Spain, the *Tarta de Santiago* rules supreme. As the one cake recipe I selected for *Start Fresh!*, this treasure is, without a doubt, one of the best almond cakes I've ever eaten. It's quick to whip up and quicker to enjoy. The good news is that it contains no butter or flour and so every bite can be enjoyed without guilt. I always keep one tucked away in the freezer. It's wonderful with summer berries from local farmers or with sliced oranges and dates.

ALMOND TART

4 large eggs, separated

1 cup (250 mL) white sugar

2¼ cups (560 mL) finely ground almonds

¼ cup (60 mL) Grand Marnier or other orange liqueur, or orange juice

ORANGE JUICE GLAZE

½ cup (125 mL) orange juice

2 Tbsp (30 mL) honey

1 or 2 drops orange blossom water (optional, available at specialty shops)

COMPOTE

5 large oranges, peeled and thinly sliced

6 large dates, thinly sliced

2 Tbsp (30 mL) coarsely chopped toasted almonds or pistachios

ground cinnamon

fresh mint leaves for garnish

CONTINUED ON NEXT PAGE

Serves 8 to 10

PER SERVING
430 calories
10 g protein
24 g fat
46 g carbohydrate
5 g fiber
26 mg sodium

Chef's Secret

ALMOND CAKES Ever wondered what gives flourless cakes their dense richness? The answer is almond meal, a finely ground meal made from blanched and then ground almonds. The natural oil in almonds adds moisture, richness and texture to cakes. Store the almond meal in the refrigerator for up to 3 months.

A FEW HOURS BEFORE Prepare the Almond Tart. Preheat the oven to 375°F (190°C). Butter and flour a 9-inch (23 cm) round cake pan and line with parchment paper. Beat the egg yolks in a large bowl. Gradually add ¾ cup (175 mL) of the sugar. Beat until creamy and light yellow, about 5 minutes. Gently fold in the ground almonds and Grand Marnier. Set aside. In a separate bowl, beat the egg whites until foamy and then gradually add the remaining ¼ cup (60 mL) sugar. Beat until stiff. Stir a little of the egg whites into the almond mixture. Gently fold in the remaining egg whites in 2 batches. Pour the batter into the prepared pan and bake about 25 to 30 minutes, or until a skewer inserted in the center of the tart comes out clean. Cool. Remove from the pan. Freeze, or leave at room temperature, wrapped well and serve over the next day or two. Sprinkle the top of the cake with icing sugar before serving. Slice in thin wedges.

Prepare the Orange Juice Glaze. Combine the orange juice and honey in a small bowl with the orange blossom water (if using). Blend well. Cover and refrigerate until ready to serve.

TO SERVE Place a slice of cake on each dessert plate. Place 2 or 3 slices of orange on 1 side of the cake. Drizzle a little of the Orange Juice Glaze over the oranges. Sprinkle a few dates and nuts over the orange slices, along with a little cinnamon. Decorate with 1 or 2 mint leaves. If you like, you could also serve it with a small scoop of orange sorbet.

LUCIA'S BANANA ICE *with* BERRY PURÉE

Low-cal ice cream? It can't be low-cal because it's so creamy and rich! But believe it. I call this my "energy revitalizer." Our granddaughter Lucia whips up a batch for us whenever she comes over for a visit. Children love it, and it's fun for them to make homemade ice cream. Whenever you have too many ripe bananas, pop them into the freezer and you have the beginnings of an instant soft ice cream to satisfy any craving, any time.

6 large ripe bananas

2 cups (500 mL) fresh or frozen unsweetened raspberries or strawberries

½ cup (125 mL) low-fat vanilla or fruit yogurt

fresh berries for garnish

1 OR 2 DAYS OR EVEN WEEKS BEFORE Peel the ripe bananas, and freeze in sealed plastic containers (bananas should be fully ripe but not dark). Allow 4 to 5 hours for them to freeze.

Purée the raspberries and strain in a fine-mesh strainer. Refrigerate, or freeze until needed and thaw overnight in the refrigerator.

JUST BEFORE SERVING Cut the frozen bananas into thin chunks and zap in a food processor with the yogurt. Whirl several minutes, stirring frequently, just until thickened and creamy. The mixture should be like soft ice cream.

TO SERVE Spoon about 2 Tbsp (30 mL) of berry purée into a wine goblet or sorbet dish, place a few spoonfuls of banana ice on top and garnish with the fresh berries.

Serves 4 to 6

PER SERVING
160 calories
2 g protein
4 g fat
34 g carbohydrate
4 g fiber
8 mg sodium

AZTEC ICE CREAM *with* LIME SAUCE

Serves 4 to 6

....

PER SERVING
156 calories
5 g protein
0 g fat
30 g carbohydrate
0 g fiber
60 mg sodium

This tantalizing ice cream "teaser" is a recipe from Chef Glenys Morgan. It was always a big hit whenever we made it for our cooking classes. It's especially refreshing with Mexican food; try it with the Tex-Mex Salmon Taco Party menu (page 55).

AZTEC ICE CREAM

4 cups (1 L) fat-free frozen yogurt or low-fat vanilla ice cream

3 Tbsp (45 mL) dark rum

1 tsp (5 mL) cinnamon

½ tsp (2 mL) red pepper flakes

LIME SAUCE

1 cup (250 mL) water

1 cup (250 mL) sugar

zest of 4 limes

4 tsp (20 mL) pure vanilla

thin slices of lime for garnish

1 OR 2 DAYS BEFORE Prepare the Aztec Ice Cream. Soften the frozen yogurt slightly in a medium-sized bowl. Fold in the rum, cinnamon and red pepper flakes. Freeze in a sealed container until ready to serve.

Prepare the Lime Sauce. Warm the water and sugar in a saucepan over low heat until the sugar is dissolved. Add the lime zest and slowly bring to a boil. Turn heat down and simmer until the zest is translucent, about 10 minutes. Remove from heat and cool to room temperature. Add the vanilla. Cover and refrigerate.

TO SERVE Put a scoop of the ice cream into a wine goblet. Drizzle the lime sauce over. Garnish with a thin slice of the lime.

JILL'S BERRIES *in* ROSÉ WINE JELLY

It was fun hosting Global TV's "Saturday Chefs" for a decade from 1991 to 2001. Jill Kropp, Global's energetic evening host, joined me for many of our TV segments. She named this bubbly dessert "The Adults' Party Jell-O." Try this whimsical dessert. It's light and low in calories (which we love).

3½ cups (875 mL) mixed fresh berries (strawberries, raspberries and blueberries)

½ cup (125 mL) water

¼ cup (60 mL) white sugar

1 Tbsp (15 mL) gelatin (1 packet)

one 6½ oz (175 mL) bottle rosé wine, or well-chilled sparkling rosé or champagne

1 cup (250 mL) raspberry or strawberry sorbet for garnish

THE DAY BEFORE Divide the mixed berries evenly among 4 martini glasses or sorbet dishes. Set aside. Combine the water and sugar in a small saucepan and stir over low heat until the sugar is dissolved. Remove from the heat, sprinkle in the gelatin and mix with a small whisk until the gelatin is dissolved. Slowly add the wine and mix just to blend. Top the 4 berry-filled glasses evenly with the wine mixture and refrigerate for least 4 hours to set.

TO SERVE Top each glass with a small scoop of berry sorbet.

Serves 4

PER SERVING
131 calories
0 g protein
0 g fat
23 g carbohydrate
4 g fiber
12 mg sodium

Chef's Secret
ROSÉ OR WHITE BUBBLY
Sparkling or flat rosé wine is an interesting alternative to the sparkling white wine, which is fun, too. You don't have to buy an expensive bubbly wine for this dessert.

Fitness and Nutrition Information Index

Recipe Index

About the Authors

DIANE CLEMENT

Diane is the author of the award-winning, bestselling *Chef on the Run* cookbook series, as well as the former chef of Tomato Fresh Food Café, which she co-owned with her actresss daughter, Jennifer. She was a sprinter on the 1956 Canadian Olympic Team and a bronze medalist at the 1958 Commonwealth Games, as well as a coach and past president of Athletics Canada and Team Manager of the Canadian Olympics Athletics Team. More recently, she was on the Board of Directors on the Bid Committee for the 2010 Olympic Games. Diane lectures internationally along with husband, Doug, on lifestyle choices—"Food, Fitness and Fun"—and hosted Global TV's "Saturday Chefs" from 1991 to 2001. Diane is a member of the International Les Dames d'Escoffier, and received the Queen's Jubilee Medal in recognition of her contribution to fitness and sport.

DR. DOUG CLEMENT

Doug is an internationally recognized sports medicine clinician and researcher who has been active as an Olympic and Commonwealth althlete and coach. Inducted into the BC Sports Hall of Fame and the Canadian Olympic Hall of Fame, he is Professor Emeritus in the Faculty of Medicine at the University of British Columbia. He is also a former team physician for the Vancouver Canucks of the National Hockey League. He has been honored with a number of academic and professional awards including the Order of Canada.

Doug and Diane are the cofounders of the successful Richmond Kajaks Athletic Club, the members of which train at the Clement Track in Richmond, BC. They also created the Achilles International Track and Field Society, which founded the Vancouver Sun Run in 1984. The Sun Run is a 10K run that promotes exercise and health. In its first year, 3,200 people participated. In 2007, that number grew to 54,000, including 1,100 corporate firms, making it one of the largest 10K runs in the world.